The Nursing Process in Psychiatric Nursing

Felicity Stockwell

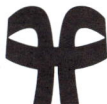

CROOM HELM

London • Sydney • Dover, New Hampshire

© 1985 Felicity Stockwell
Croom Helm Ltd, Provident House, Burrell Row,
Beckenham, Kent BR3 1AT

Croom Helm Australia Pty Ltd, Suite 4, 6th Floor,
64-76 Kippax Street, Surry Hills, NSW 2010, Australia

British Library Cataloguing in Publication Data

Stockwell, Felicity
   The nursing process in psychiatric nursing.
   1. Psychiatric nursing
  I. Title
   610.73′68   RC440

   ISBN 0-7099-3311-8

Croom Helm, 51 Washington Street,
Dover, Hew Hampshire 03820, USA

Library of Congress Cataloging in Publication Data

Stockwell, Felicity
   The nursing process in psychiatric nursing.
   Includes bibliographies and index.
   1. Psychiatric nursing. I. Title.
[DNLM: 1. Nursing Process. 2. Psychiatric Nursing.
WY 160 S866n]
RC440.S78   1985   610.73′68   85-9673

   ISBN 0-7099-3311-8 (pbk.)

Photoset in English Times by Pat and Anne Murphy,
Printed and bound in Great Britain by Mackays of Chatham Ltd, Kent

CONTENTS

TO

HELEN AND JUDITH

ACKNOWLEDGEMENTS

I should like to thank those members of staff and patients at Whittingham Hospital who have helped me with ideas and encouragement. I would also like to thank my colleagues in the School of Nursing who have given their time and effort to reading the script and offering constructive criticism, Mrs Sheila Payne and Mrs Brenda Cooke for their patient help with typing the manuscript, and, especially my family for their encouragement and co-operation over many months.

INTRODUCTION

This book is written specifically for nurses working with mentally ill patients, both in hospital and in the community. There are, already, many books available about the Nursing Process and it should be possible for mental nurses to gain information and understanding from them, because there is a common core to nursing practice that applies to both general and mental nursing, and all patients share a common humanity. However, there are enough differences for legislation to provide for separate training and qualifying examinations for general and mental nursing and, in practice, the day-to-day work differs in both the emphasis and the activities.

The book is a personal interpretation of many authors' contributions to understanding and implementing the Nursing Process. It is essentially practical in its approach and related to the realities of mental nursing at the present time, while bearing in mind the shift towards community-based rather than institutional care.

There may be readers who are wondering why a book entitled *The Nursing Process in Psychiatric Nursing* is referring to mental nurses and mental nursing. This is because legislation refers to and recognises mental nurses, while common usage almost always uses the term psychiatric nurses (and 'psychy' secondment from general training!). Thus I am not specifically addressing the subject of mental handicap in this book, although hopefully it will prove useful to nurses in this field. From 'attendants on the insane', via 'mental nurses' and 'mental illness nurses' to 'psychiatric nurses', the names have changed and the care has evolved. Because the majority of available textbooks use the term psychiatric nursing in their titles and context and the term has come into common parlance, it will be used for the remainder of the book.

On a personal note, and with apologies to many other interpreters of the Nursing Process, readers will find very little mention of problems or a problem-solving approach in the following pages. I am not suggesting there is no problem-solving element in psychiatric nursing, but where it becomes the focus of identifying what nursing a particular patient needs there is a tendency to concentrate on the patient's pathology to the exclusion of other aspects of the patient's behaviour. Were I to be admitted, I would want the team to get to know me for whatever strengths and worth I was clinging on to, and then to understand and help my difficulties, rather than find myself regarded as a package of problems.

Hopefully, because the book requires readers to think and work on the different aspects of the Nursing Process as they read it, at the end if anyone feels that a 'problem-solving' approach is the most appropriate they will have gained enough information to incorporate it and adapt their documentation to it.

There is another area where I diverge from other interpreters of the Nursing Process philosophy and this concerns the aspect of individualising nursing care. For many writers this requires assigning a nurse to carry out the nursing and be responsible for a particular patient or group of patients. Many psychiatric wards have very small teams of nurses and sometimes some of them are unqualified and the turnover of nurses, especially in training wards, is often more rapid than the turnover of patients, many of whom may be long-stay. These factors mean that sometimes the only possible and practical way of assigning the nursing care is for the Sister to use task allocation. Yet with thoughtful attention to the tasks to be done, the nurses available and the individual patients' needs, it should be possible to prevent the routinised, autocratic and hierarchical system sometimes observed in psychiatric wards, that is felt to be a factor that prevents nurses knowing their patients as whole people.

There is also the possibility that the group dynamics in a ward can be realistic and therapeutic tools whereby patients can learn from their experiments and experiences about their strengths and difficulties in relation to others. Many mentally ill people have difficulties in this area and the fact that we feel more valuable when others choose to spend time with us rather than when we feel they have to do so can be used as a very useful tool. However this is true only where there is freedom of interaction and patients are not referring to 'my nurse' and nurses are not talking about 'my patient'.

It is shown in the book that individualisation is achieved by encouraging the patients' participation in the care planning and by ensuring that each patient receives the nursing care appropriate to his or her particular needs in the context of the group as a whole. There will be occasions when it is useful to appoint a named nurse as a 'key-worker' with an individual patient, but this would be specifically planned.

Throughout the book I have taken it for granted that psychiatric nurses are knowledgeable about psychiatric nursing, but because implementing the Nursing Process needs the ability to use some particular nursing skills, these have been reviewed in some detail in the appropriate chapters.

Finally, a word of warning: this is not a recipe book that will provide straightforward usable solutions to implementing the Nursing Process. Rather, it is a tourist guide that will encourage active thinking, exploration and experiment and, hopefully, lead with perseverance to the rewards of achievement.

1 THE NURSING PROCESS — WHAT IS IT?

At its simplest the Nursing Process is a systematic way of consciously thinking about patients or clients, ensuring that what each patient needs in the way of nursing care is identified, organising and doing the nursing, checking and recording that the required nursing has been carried out, and evaluating the effectiveness of the nursing care given.

At this point you can probably feel this book is not for you as you probably do that already. So what is different about the Nursing Process?

The reading list at the end of this chapter refers to a selection of various books that define and explain the Nursing Process. The aim of this book is to share in an accessible way these ideas and understandings and to present them as they can relate to psychiatric nursing.

So we will define the Nursing Process again.

It is a *systematic* way of *consciously* thinking about patients or clients, ensuring that what *each* patient needs in the way of nursing is *identified*, organising and doing the nursing, checking and *recording* that the required nursing has been carried out, and *evaluating* the effectiveness of the care given.

Now let us explore the emphasised words in the context of current nursing practice.

First of all *systematic*. A system is defined as 'a whole composed of parts in orderly arrangement according to some scheme or plan'.

A definition of *process* is 'a continuous and regular succession of actions carried on in a definite manner'.

These two definitions applied to nursing would see it as an ongoing activity, carried out according to a plan, in orderly stages.

The opposite of 'systematic' is 'chaotic' and no one would or could say that psychiatric nursing is chaotic. However, it is important that the word 'systematic' is being applied to the activity of nursing and not to the tasks of nursing. Many nursing tasks are carried out systematically and the system can become very inflexible, and is then called a routine — or even a ritual. Where routines or rituals form the basis of nursing practice it is likely that where a patient's needs are not being met by the 'routine' he will present with problem behaviour which the nursing staff will then 'manage'. This has been called 'crisis management' or 'trouble-shooting nursing', but is what I call 'expediency nursing' because it calls for snap decisions based on limited information and refers not only to crises but to all sorts of more trivial nursing interventions.

The 'system' of the Nursing Process sees the overall activity of nursing as having a series of identifiable stages which require a succession of actions to be carried out.

These stages are:

(1) *Assessment* of the patient and their nursing requirements.
(2) *Planning* what nursing care can and should be carried out.
(3) *Drawing up instructions* for the nursing care of the patient, based on the plan (sometimes called nursing prescription or orders).
(4) *Implementing*, or carrying out the nursing instructions.
(5) *Evaluating* to what extent the nursing activities have been helpful, or otherwise, and re-assessing the patient and planning further care as necessary.

These stages of the system are carried out in sequence, but the evaluation leads to the re-assessment of the patient and further planning, implementation and evaluation until the patient no longer needs nursing care.

The next word to be emphasised is *consciously*. This word embodies the most exacting aspect of the Nursing Process because it requires that the nurse not only makes conscious, but also puts into words for speaking and writing, much that by habit is given no attention.

The first stage of the Nursing Process is assessment and for good planning it requires more information about patients than is usually available or communicated. The ability to describe patients in the here and now, with an account of their strengths and disabilities and their endearing or less endearing characteristics, without communicating individual value judgements, is what is required. It needs not only good observation skills but also a conscious effort to overcome the normal principles of perception by which we always discount much of what is available for seeing, hearing and feeling.

The other aspect of care that has to be made conscious is the decision-making process that determines what nursing action should be taken and why. Sometimes the decision is influenced by medical policy, rules, rituals or routines, but even within these bounds there is often choice as to how or which particular nursing intervention is carried out. There is also in psychiatric nursing a larger or lesser part of the day where the nursing team has the responsibility and the self-determination to decide what nursing to do, or maybe not to do. It should be possible to put into words why one action rather than another was decided upon, instead of explaining it as hunch or intuition.

We now come to the *each*. The Nursing Process is frequently described as an individualised approach to nursing care and is often interpreted as meaning that a certain patient or patients are allocated to a particular nurse or team of nurses for their nursing care. This might be an ideal and practicable in the community setting, but in the majority of institutional psychiatric nursing situations it is an impossible ideal. It is not, however, a barrier to implementing the Nursing Process. When the definition refers to *each* patient it means that the aim of the nursing team should be to know each and every patient in their care well enough to know his likes and dislikes, his strengths and weaknesses, and his special characteristics. Thus decisions about allocating the nursing care meet the priorities for nursing *each* patient and ensure that every patient gets an appropriate share of nursing time during every shift.

Each also means that wherever possible the patient should be consulted about his viewpoint, his feelings and his ideas about the care he needs.

Many wards have a few patients who merge into the background because routine provision seems to meet their needs and they make no demands on the staff. They may well be content and appear to be functioning at their best, but the Nursing Process philosophy means that someone should spend some time interacting with the patient to ensure that this is so. An individual approach to nursing care does not mean that group activities should not be carried out, but it does mean that every member participating in a group session is there because it is suitable and beneficial for them at that time, and not just because it is convenient.

Identifying what nursing care each patient needs is emphasised because although it might sound self-evident and easy it is in fact proving to be very difficult to pin-point particular nursing requirements and put them into words without using jargon or meaningless generalisations. The same comment applies to *recording* nursing instructions and *evaluation* of nursing actions and these difficulties are given detailed consideration later in this book.

For now suffice it to say that all these stages require specific skills that initially have to be learnt and then constantly practised. However, it is important to stress that at the 'point of delivery' there is nothing magical about the Nursing Process that it is going to improve or detract from the quality and the expertise of any nursing care any individual nurse carries out. That is, no amount of 'doing the Nursing Process' will, for example, make a nurse who is a skilled listener less able to listen, nor will it turn an impatient nurse into a patient one. However, if the philosophy of the Nursing Process is influencing the team's care, then the nursing is more likely to be appropriate and monitored, and as a result overall standards of care could improve.

Suggested Further Reading

Heath, J., and Law, G. M. *Nursing Process. What is it?* Adapted for psychiatric nursing by Ivan Cross (NHS Learning Resources Unit, Sheffield, 1983)

Irving, S. *Basic Psychiatric Nursing*, Chapter 9 (W. B. Saunders Co., Philadelphia, 1983)

Kratz, C. R. (ed.) *The Nursing Process* (Bailliere Tindall, London, 1979)

Long, R. *Systematic Nursing Care* (Faber and Faber, London, 1981)

McFarlane of Llandaff and Castledine, G. *The Practice of Nursing Using the Nursing Process* (Blackwell Scientific Publications, Oxford, 1982)

Sundeen, S. J., Stuart, G. W., Rankin, E. D. and Cohen, S. A. *Nurse-Client Interaction. Implementing the Nursing Process*, 2nd edn (C. V. Mosby Co., St Louis, 1981)

Ward, M. *The Nursing Process in Psychiatry* (Churchill Livingstone, Edinburgh, 1984)

2 PHILOSOPHIES, MODELS AND CONCEPTS OF PSYCHIATRIC NURSING

Many attempts have been made to define nursing, to describe nursing and to construct models of nursing. Whether these exercises have been carried out as a theoretical task, as an attempt to measure patients' dependency levels, as a requirement for evaluating standards of nursing care or for curriculum planning for nurse training, none of them satisfies everybody across the whole field of nursing. The truism that 'nursing is what nurses do' is a convenient side-step that evades the challenge of definition and explains nothing, but allows nurses to rest comfortably with the knowledge that as long as they are doing what they were trained to do, they are nursing and that is what nursing is.

This book is about psychiatric nursing — about its proven development and practice but also about shortcomings that could be improved with change. It is not its purpose to determine to what extent psychiatric nursing differs from or is similar to general nursing. Suffice it to say that psychiatric nursing has been regarded as different enough to warrant a separate training and register of qualified nurses and yet there must be sufficient common ground for the definition of 'nurse' to apply to both fields.

Psychiatric nursing could be said to have been first identified as a separate calling in 1885 when the first edition of the *Handbook for Attendants on the Insane* was published. The introduction to this book said it was 'designed to aid attendants to carry out the orders of the physicians' and these would be orders designed to safely contain and control 'lunatics'. Time has brought changes in the treatment and nursing care of those who are now termed 'mentally ill'. Now the role of the mental illness nurse approximates more closely to the role of the general nurse in that the psychiatrists need nurses to support and care for patients while their prescribed treatment takes effect and to care fully for patients when their treatment is of limited or of no avail. There are, however, essential differences that will always remain because of the different effects that mental illnesses have compared with physical illnesses.

As psychiatric nurses know, caring for mentally ill patients calls for a range of activities, with some patients being very physically dependent on the nursing team while others need mainly the psychological interventions that are their special skill. However, because the ratio of mentally ill patients over the age of 65 (geriatric, by DHSS definition) is high, some examples in the text are purposefully chosen so that nurses in psychogeriatric wards can feel the book has relevance to their sphere of work.

The Nursing Process aims to make the practice of nursing systematic and conscious and for many nurses this means changing some habits of a nursing lifetime. For change to occur it requires some awareness of the present state of affairs and some dissatisfaction with it and an understanding that the remedy can lie within one's own actions and is not entirely dependent on more staff or more resources. Change needs an open mind and a willingness actively to think and question. As you read this chapter you are asked to read it slowly and strive towards answering the questions raised, as honestly as you can, as they relate to you.

The first question is 'What do you, as a psychiatric nurse, do or expect others to do?'

You may be a staff nurse, an experienced charge nurse, a nursing officer, a clinical teacher, or in any other role in which you are employed because you are a Registered Mental Nurse. Whether you are working directly with patients, as a manager enabling others to nurse, or teaching others to nurse, you must know what nurses do or are expected to do in relation to your sphere of responsibility.

Try and make conscious as much as you can and then write it down. It is important to avoid such generalised terms as 'caring for' or 'looking after' or any of their synonyms and you may well find it is not as easy a task as it sounds . . .

When you have answered this first question, you have identified, at least in part, what the job of nursing is. Now you can move to the next question which will lead you to explore the philosophy of psychiatric nursing. Philosophy in this context is used to mean the attitudes, values and wisdom that we hold that influence the way we act.

The second question asks 'Why do you do psychiatric nursing?'

It is often easier to make judgements about other people's attitudes and values from our observations of their behaviour than it is to make conscious these aspects in ourselves. Individual philosophies can range from the very cynical to the extremely altruistic, with the majority coming somewhere between. They can be influenced by religious beliefs, cultural context and political commitment. They are formed through experience, but once formed are not easily modified by experience.

Phil

An individual's philosophy will influence the way he behaves. By describing two different ways of behaving in the same situation it is likely you will make value judgements of the motivating philosophies and this can help to make consious your own attitudes and values and help to answer this second question.

The example is a ward for long-stay, fairly independent, ageing patients. The first person in charge of such a ward states that she only comes to work for the money and her superannuation rights. She ensures the patients are kept fed and watered, clean and dry but feels it is unkind and a waste of time to make any more demands on them. Office work can expand to fill the day and providing you 'keep your nose clean' there is no hassle from the bosses, and you certainly get no thanks for doing any more.

The second person also keeps her patients fed and watered and clean and dry, but brings a cake from home for a resident's birthday, constantly chivvies the nursing officers to get more rails in the toilets and new pictures on the walls, has eye-to-eye contact and chats with all the residents daily and uses imagination to inspire the team members to enhance the residents experience because 'nothing is too much trouble for our patients'.

You have already made value judgements about those two accounts. Make them conscious and relate them to your own feelings and ideals and if you can capture *why* you feel some parts are 'right' or 'wrong', useful or less useful and can identify *why* you would do it differently, you are possibly nearer to being able to write down what your attitudes and feelings are towards the people in your care and the colleagues you work with and thus define your philosophy of nursing . . .

Having identified, at least in some measure, your philosophy of nursing, the most difficult question now has to be posed and this is 'How do you do psychiatric nursing?' A possible answer to this question could be 'by intuition' and there is no doubt that many nursing decisions are arrived at unconsciously, and others are carried out routinely. However, for the nursing process to act as a systematic means of individualising and improving care it is essential to be able to make conscious and identify the range of choices from which the most useful will be implemented, in all aspects of nursing.

Being able to identify how you decide what nursing to do only answers the question posed in part. Deciding when to implement the care and for how long to carry it on, is another component of nursing, but the most difficult aspect to identify is what it is of nursing that makes it a skilled, purposeful and helpful activity that is more than the sum of the tasks that have to be done.

Because nursing is so complex it is extremely difficult to find words to make adequate sense of it. Attempts to do this have been made, mainly in America, mainly by 'academics' and at the time of writing related, primarily, to general nursing. These attempts to make sense of nursing have resulted in a variety of 'conceptual models of nursing care'.

Models are simplified representations of larger or more complicated things and 'conceptual' models are simplified expressions of complex ideas, usually summarised in the form of a chart. Readers who are familiar with models of nursing or who wish to explore the topic in more depth are referred to the reading list at the end of this chapter. For others who may be on more unfamiliar ground, with due apology to their originators, there follows, in a simplified form, an outline of some of the more commonly referred to models of nursing with illustration of how they can influence nursing practice.

The models selected are those which have had, or still have, application in psychiatric hospitals and will probably be recognisable to many readers.

For an example of a situation needing nursing intervention that can be related to the models of care described, let us take an elderly lady, in hospital for many years with a diagnosis of schizophrenia, who over recent weeks has become intermittently incontinent. She is distressed when found to be wet, but otherwise shows no appreciable change in her mental state.

A Medical Model of Nursing

This model sees the patient as someone who is diagnosed as having a defined illness and sees the nurse as the eyes and ears of the doctor, observing the patient in his absence, and as the hands of the doctor, carrying out prescribed treatment and providing care and safety for the patient until treatment is effective.

The intermittent incontinence of our example will be viewed by this model as either a symptom of the patient's mental illness or as a pathology of ageing. The nurse's initial response is likely to be to report the matter to the doctor for investigation and possible prescription. Medical intervention may, in a few cases, cure the incontinence. If, however, it does not, it will be regarded as inevitable and will be managed in whatever way has become 'routine' in that particular ward.

A Problem-solving Model of Nursing

This model sees the patient as having an illness that interferes with some, or many, aspects of living, thus producing problems in managing life satisfactorily. It sees the nurse as skilled in identifying the patient's problems and having a repertoire of nursing actions to solve or alleviate the problems.

The intermittent incontinence will be seen as a problem on both physical and social grounds. Physical, because of damage to the patient's skin, possible infection and perhaps an accident through slipping in 'puddles' on the floor; social, because of the smell being offensive and furniture and clothes spoilt.

The 'problem' in this case may take time to be recognised because the occasional 'accident' may not be regarded as a problem, but once it is recognised, the solution is likely to be regular reminders to visit the toilet. This strategy will often solve the problem, although not always, especially if the cause of the incontinence is other than a decreasing awareness of when the bladder is full, or a physical slowing down, preventing reaching the toilet in time. Where the strategy fails, the incontinence is likely to be seen as an insoluble problem and again be managed in a routine way.

A Needs-meeting Model of Nursing

This model sees the patient as a bio-social system whose healthy functioning is dependent on physiological, psycho-social and spiritual needs being met. Illness can prevent or inhibit the meeting of some of these needs. It sees the nurse as an agent who uses skills to identify where needs are not being met and who has the ability to ensure the needs are met or can assist the patient to compensate for any lack.

With reference to our patient with intermittent incontinence, some writers would regard elimination and excretion as 'needs', while others would see them as functions and would regard incontinence as threatening or not meeting the needs for safety and dignity. Whichever the viewpoint, with the 'needs' model of nursing the patient will be seen as needing regular toileting, carried out in privacy and needing observation and care of the skin and pressure areas.

An Activities of Daily Living Model of Nursing

A list of the Activities of Daily Living is but a list until someone states how she sees the patient being affected with regard to them and how the nurse's interventions relate to them. There are several models of nursing based on Activities of Daily Living (or Fundamental Human Needs, as a similar list is identified).

In the United Kingdom, Nancy Roper and her colleagues have had publicised what has come to be known as the 'Roper' model of nursing. This model sees the patient as being on a continuum between dependence and independence for each of the listed Activities of Daily Living, and sees the nurse as preserving as far as possible the patient's usual (healthy) habits associated with each Activity of Living and any nursing interventions as having a 'preventing' a 'comforting' or a 'dependent' component, or a mixture of these.

This model would see the intermittent incontinence of the example as the patient not 'eliminating' in the usual way and tending towards 'dependency' for the 'elimination' Activity of Living. It would see the nurse as assisting the patient to get to the toilet in time or discreetly managing the incontinence with appropriate means, and in so doing drawing on each of the 'preventing', 'dependent' and 'comforting' components of nursing skills.

It will perhaps be evident when reading these synopses of models of nursing that in practice it is possible to recognise nursing based on several of the models. Whatever seems most familiar on reading about them, it is likely that all these models have had a significant influence on the way in which the nursing process has been implemented in general nursing. However, psychiatric nurses may well recognise a deficiency in all these models.

In answer to the first two questions of this chapter it is probable that a commitment to encouraging patients to do as much for themselves as possible figures high on the list of what psychiatric nurses do. For many years it has been a prescription for preventing or treating institutionalisation, that, as far as possible, patients be helped and encouraged to accept responsibility for their own welfare and occupation and be as independent as their disabilities allow. In part this independence is increased by having realistic decision-making opportunities planned into the day.

From their original preventative aspect these factors have come to be seen as fundamental in enhancing the patient's feelings of uniqueness and worth. They are seen as essential commitments to care, going further than the 'individualising of care' that is part of the philosophy of the Nursing Process.

For this reason a more appropriate nursing model is needed in the psychiatric field. The following account is of a model that has evolved following discussions about psychiatric nursing, especially in relation to setting up pilot studies for implementing the Nursing Process. Called an 'enhancement' model of nursing care it is proferred as a concept that might prove acceptable or might act as a stimulus to new ideas and other models.

An Enhancement Model of Psychiatric Nursing

This model sees the patient as a person with many innate and learned capacities and who, through living, has grown, developed and learned many skills and aptitudes, but who through suffering from mental illness becomes dependent, to some degree, on the help, support and care of others. It sees the nurse as a person who primarily identifies the strengths and capabilities of the patient and devises strategies and opportunities to ensure these are exercised and enhanced. Secondarily she uses skills to alleviate or minimise difficulties and disabilities, while supporting the patient during whatever psychiatric treatment he may be having.

A diagram of this model is shown in Figure 2.1 and a fuller account and explanation is given in Appendix 2.

To illustrate the influence of this model of care on nursing practice the same account of the patient with intermittent

Figure 2.1: An Enhancement Model of Psychiatric Nursing

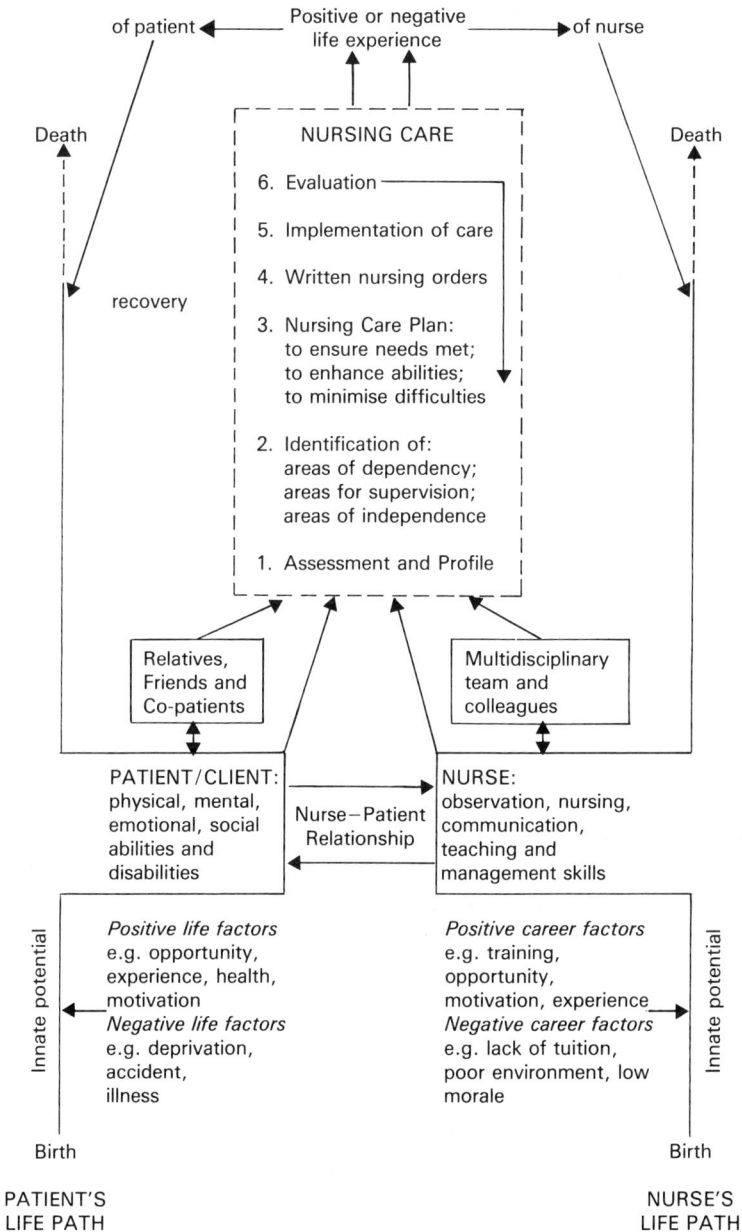

of patient ◄——— Positive or negative ———► of nurse
                      life experience

Death   Death

- -
| NURSING CARE |
| |
| 6. Evaluation ───────────── |
5. Implementation of care	
4. Written nursing orders	
recovery	
3. Nursing Care Plan:	
to ensure needs met;	
to enhance abilities;   ▼
to minimise difficulties
2. Identification of:
areas of dependency;
areas for supervision;
areas of independence
1. Assessment and Profile
- -

┌─────────────────┐   ┌─────────────────┐
│ Relatives,   │   │ Multidisciplinary│
│ Friends and   │   │ team and   │
│ Co-patients   │   │ colleagues   │
└─────────────────┘   └─────────────────┘

PATIENT/CLIENT: NURSE:
physical, mental,   observation, nursing,
emotional, social   Nurse–Patient   communication,
abilities and   Relationship   teaching and
disabilities   management skills

Innate potential

Positive life factors   *Positive career factors*
e.g. opportunity,   e.g. training,
experience, health,   opportunity,
motivation   motivation, experience
Negative life factors   *Negative career factors*
e.g. deprivation,   e.g. lack of tuition,
accident,   poor environment, low
illness   morale

Innate potential

Birth   Birth

PATIENT'S   NURSE'S
LIFE PATH   LIFE PATH

incontinence will be used. Focusing on the patient's strengths, the first nursing strategy would be to observe discreetly the successful visits to the toilet. When it is accurately established how well and in what circumstances the patient manages to be continent it is likely to be easier to identify the cause of the occasional incontinence.

In an actual such incident, after a programme of 'reminding' had not solved the problem and had made the patient hostile and abusive it was agreed to observe her when visiting the toilet for a few days. It was noticed that she always went first to a particular cubicle, but if this was occupied went into the next one. If both were occupied she 'had an accident'. When she was in the second cubicle it was noticed there was no 'noise' and a discreet look under the door revealed the patient standing over the bowl. Being short-legged her knickers were in the way and got wet. The differences between the two toilet cubicles was that there were handrails in the first one but not in the other and the problem turned out to be not incontinence but increasing age causing lack of balance and confidence and the occasional incontinence was remedied by putting handrails in all the toilets.

The example that has been used above to illustrate the various models is essentially a physical nursing problem. Therefore further illustration of the application of an enhancement model of care where the problems are more psychological is given below.

Let us take the case of a man brought in for admission by his concerned wife. He shows psycho-motor retardation, expresses feelings of guilt and unworthiness and states it would be better for all if he were dead.

For many nurses this would be enough information for the team to decide how to nurse this particular patient. Basing practice on an enhancement model of nursing the team would chat to the wife about her husband, eliciting information about his strengths and abilities before his illness. The assessment interview would focus on what he can and, if anything, wishes to do at the present, or whether there is anything the nursing team can offer that he could imagine would make life more tolerable in the here and now — for example, solitude or listening to some particular music. Within the limits of his present functioning it would explore his past achievements and accentuate the skills and abilities he must have had to make a happy home, do a responsible job or whatever is appropriate. The plan of care will then take into account any of the positive aspects that have been identified.

Not all problems have clear-cut solutions, but very often accurate identification of the causative factors and clues to the best intervention can be found by directed observation and attentive listening.

The diagram of the 'enhancement model of nursing care' in Figure 2.1 illustrates the essential interaction of the positive aspects of the patient and the nurse that determines what care the patient needs and ensures the effectiveness of what is carried out. At its most optimistic the partnership works towards the experience of suffering from mental illness enhancing the patient's life so that he functions the better for having been ill, or at its most pessimistic, ensuring the highest quality of life within a continuing-care environment.

It is because psychiatric nursing puts an emphasis on patients doing as much for themselves as they can, encourages them to preserve their identity and individuality and plays down the 'patient role' as far as possible, that there is a particular need for a specific 'Nursing Process' book. By now it should be evident that what motivates the individual and the nursing team, and how they use and share their expertise, will influence not only current practice, but also how accepting they are of, and how adaptable they are to innovation.

Having read this far, the reader should have given active consideration to her personal views on the nature of psychiatric nursing and the part she plays in providing care. For those who have not been able to put this down in writing, the author has offered her personal answers to the questions posed and these are set out in Appendix 1.

The following chapters take each stage of the nursing process, identify the particular knowledge needed and examine the skills required. They explore their practical application amd make some suggestions, but they do not claim to offer any 'recipes' for 'doing' the Nursing Process.

Eventually, it might be possible to use documentation others have developed. However, at the time of writing it is still a necessary discipline to devise or modify record-keeping documents so that they are appropriate for the particular patients being cared for. In this way they serve the nursing team and do not become its master by demanding too much time and effort to complete.

Suggested Further Reading

Aggleton, P., and Chalmers, H. 'Models and theories.' 1. Defining the terms. 2. The Roy Adaptation Model. 3. The Riehl Interaction Model. 4. Rogers Unitary Field Model. 5. The Orem Self-care Model. 6. Roper's Activities of Living Model. 7. Henderson's Model. *Nursing Times*, Vol. 80, No's 36, 40, 45, 50, Vol. 81, No's 1, 7, 10 (1984/5)

Griffith, J. W., and Christenson, P. J. *Nursing Process, Application of Theories, Frameworks and Models* (C. V. Mosby, St Louis, 1982)

Henderson, V. *Basic Principles of Nursing Care* (International Council of Nurses, Geneva, 1969)

Riehl, J. P., and Roy, C. *Conceptual Models for Nursing Practice*, 2nd edn (Appleton-Century-Crofts, New York, 1980)

Roper, N., Logan, W. W., and Tierney, A. J. (eds) *The Elements of Nursing* (1980), *Learning to Use the Process of Nursing* (1981), *Using a Model for Nursing* (1983), (Churchill Livingstone, Edinburgh)

3 ASSESSMENT: GETTING TO KNOW THE PATIENT

Assessment is the means by which the nurse gets to know the patient and his problems and it has to be the foundation on which all nursing care is planned. Sources of information about the patient as a unique person in need of nursing care come from looking at and listening to the patient and from various tests. This is called primary information. There are also data from documents, accounts from relatives and friends and information obtained by other members of the multidisciplinary team; this is called secondary information.

Assessments must be recorded in a way that enables a nurse new to the ward to identify patients and gain a picture of their current personality and behaviour, their strengths and their difficulties, and their likes and dislikes. To be effective, assessments must serve the purpose of identifying what nursing care the patient needs. They must therefore indicate those areas in which the patient needs not only help and support, but also encouragement and supervision, and where he can safely contribute and manage for himself.

As part of normal social behaviour, whenever we meet people we assess them, make a value judgement about them and modify our behaviour towards them accordingly. This process takes place at an unconscious level and usually it is only when we make judgements towards the extremes of liking or disliking that they intrude into consciousness. Assessment as a tool for planning nursing care requires that the nurse is aware of making both hasty judgements and subjective value judgements and tries to make them conscious so as to be in a better position to modify the 'normal' pattern of response. The holds true for 'reflex' responses to nice patients, but is especially important when the patient presents himself in a way that makes people feel angry, helpless, disgusted or any other negative emotion. Recognition of negative feelings should not be a cause for guilt, but should act as a cue for the nurse to seek more contact with the patient and devise opportunities to explore for hidden strengths and capabilities.

Knowledge Needed for Assessment

The knowledge required for assessment can be summarised as:

(1) An awareness and understanding of the principles of perception and how they influence what we see, hear and feel.
(2) Enough knowledge of psychology, human biology, psychopathology and physical pathology, to give meaning to what is perceived in patients and their environment.
(3) Knowledge of the law, as it relates to documentation of information about patients being a legal record, and professional responsibility for the confidentiality of the information obtained.

Skills Needed for the Assessment of Patients

These fall into four categories: observational skills; questioning skills; listening skills; and recording skills. These will now be reviewed in greater detail.

(1) Observational Skills

The ability to use sight, hearing and feeling to notice and give meaning to facts is a learned skill and what any individual nurse observes about her patients will depend on the quality of her initial learning and the degree to which she has kept the skill exercised. As with all skills, if active observation is not practised, the ability will be lost and in nursing it is sometimes the case that inferences are drawn and decisions made on very limited evidence. All facts noticed should leave a skilled observer with a question in her mind that encourages further exploration or leads to focusing on a different aspect of the patient's behaviour. The following example illustrates how a 'cue' behaviour can be observed differently by nurses with a different focus of attention and different abilities.

'On being asked to come for a bath a disorientated elderly lady in an assessment ward says she wants to play whist.'

The first nurse, concentrating on the bath and what she must notice about the patient's physical state, does not hear the request. For her it is 'background noise' and it does not reach conscious awareness.

A second nurse has the patient's 'mental state' in the foreground of her perceptions, hears the request but knows that demented patients can't play whist, and makes a joke about getting the cards wet in the bath.

A third nurse, preoccupied with what to do to keep the patients occupied during the long afternoon, on hearing the request suggests playing cards later on, thinking that even if she can't manage whist she might manage something simpler.

A fourth nurse, knowing she has to contribute to the assessment profile of this patient, uses the mention of whist to explore the patient's memories of playing whist in the past. By feigning ignorance explores her knowledge of cards and the rules of whist while bathing her, and as a result of listening will have a fair idea of whether it would be useful to produce a pack of cards.

This illustrates four possible responses to a behaviour that, as a cue for assessment, was observed and used differently in each case and indicates how differently the incident would be reported or recorded by each nurse. The example also illustrates how the Assessment stage of the Nursing Process can and should be used for a positive and beneficial interaction that builds a bridge of mutual trust and sets the standard for subsequent nursing care.

Observation is made up of first noticing what there is to be noticed as fact, and secondly giving meaning to and evaluating the facts. Observation also implies action, although one of the choices of action may be to do nothing!

All sensory information requires that we experience or feel it and then act on it, but our brain does not require that all stimuli reaching it be given attention or significance. Indeed, if this were the case we would be so overloaded that we would stop functioning. However, to be skilled observers it is necessary to know where to direct attention and consciously monitor the information received. If this is not done then the inferences and value judgements that we make in response to our perceptions at a subconscious level are what will be given voice if required. It is especially important to remember that attention must be directed to non-verbal signals as well as more obvious behaviour patterns and speech in order to make an accurate evaluation.

An example of poor observation is the sort of report on a newly admitted patient that says 'He is a nice man. Obviously depressed, but won't be any trouble'.

Where factual observations are not available then descriptions have to be in terms of subjective feelings or hunches and these often reveal as much about the observer as the observed. The ability to be aware of and communicate fact rather than value judgements and inferences is one of the many exacting disciplines of the Nursing Process philosophy. Hunches and intuition can sometimes be valid and indeed a nurse's feelings about a patient when expressed as such can be useful. However, laziness can sometimes lead to their unwitting habitual use and this is not adequate for sound nursing practice.

Having learned and practised the skill of noticing and recalling a multitude of facts about the patients, the nurse must also be able to distinguish between what is useful information and what is less relevant, and between what are likely to be useful lines of further enquiry and what less fruitful. This aspect of observation has to be based on sound knowledge and experience and is very difficult to teach. It is also difficult to evaluate to what extent any particular nurse is competent in this respect. When the assessment of patients has to be delegated to learner nurses it is tempting, when planning the documentation, to rely on lengthy itemised 'questionnaires' to make sure nothing important is left out. In some respects such forms negate the philosophy of the Nursing Process, as they tend to ritualise the gathering of information rather than providing opportunity for free expression, and focusing on what is important to the patient.

Different formats for recording assessment observations are explored in Chapter 8, but the result should be a written factual account that includes a general profile of the patient, his strengths and weaknesses, any nursing needs or problems identified and any major likes or dislikes, knowledge of which will influence the patient's stay in hospital.

(2) Questioning Skills

It might seem impertinent to suggest that grown-up people need to be taught how to ask questions. We all have an innate curiosity, but, depending on experience, this can remain active or can become dormant.

The ability to gain information and understanding about patients through questioning them has two aspects, both of which are skills that have to be learnt. The first is knowing what to ask about and the second is knowing how to ask it.

Being aware of what information is needed for safe and efficient care has priority. However, the philosophy of the Nursing Process also requires the nurse to be aware of what information it is useful to enquire about, record and share with the nursing team to enable them to know and understand the patient as a unique individual and plan more comprehensive and relevant nursing care.

Deciding what to ask about will, to some extent, be decided by the format of the assessment document but the amount of information gained will depend in large measure on the way the questions are phrased. For example, nurses are required to fill in the space beside 'Religion . . .' for all patients and routinely the question is usually phrased 'Religion?' or 'What is your religion?' with the answer being Church of England, Hindu, none or whatever. This is all right for face sheet information, but the Nursing Process philosophy dictates that the nurse should explore in detail any area that might be important, so this topic will be used to illustrate the various types of questions.

Types of Questions. There are five basic types of question.

(i) *Closed questions.* This sort of question can usually be answered with a yes or no or a single word or phrase. The question 'Religion?' or 'Any religion?' calls for a yes or no answer but often in practice gets the basic information required.

(ii) *Open or free response questions.* This type of question allows the person answering to focus on what is important to him and to reveal as much or as little as he wishes. For our example the nurse might ask 'What, if any, religious beliefs or practices do you hold or like to carry out?' The answer may well need further questions, but it provides a stimulus for possibly useful information to be revealed.

(iii) *Reflective questions.* As the word suggests, this sort of question is not used as a 'starter', but to encourage the respondent to enlarge on or clarify what he has been saying. It can often be used to explore how the patient feels about what he is saying. The answer to the question 'Do you have any religious beliefs?' might be 'Not any more' and a reflective question could be 'Any more?' or 'What do you mean, any more?' and that might throw light on past religious practice. Alternatively, the nurse could ask 'Does that bother you?' or 'How do you feel about that?' and this explores the patient's present position with regard to religion.

(iv) *Leading questions.* These questions are phrased so that it is difficult to answer in any other than an expected way. To some extent the question 'What is your religion?' is a leading question as it presupposes the respondent has a religion. However, if the patient replies 'Put down C of E, but I wouldn't say I was anything really', an example of a leading question arising from that would be 'Well, you won't want to go to Church on Sunday then, will you?' People do not have to answer leading questions in response to the lead, but learned politeness usually persuades them to 'go along' by answering in the expected way even though they may not mean it.

(v) *Sarcastic questions.* Sarcasm is designed to change another person's behaviour when that behaviour is annoying or challenging. It is a socially acceptable way of relieving frustration and is often effective in doing this. It can sometimes result in changing another person's behaviour, but this is unlikely to be the case where the problems have brought someone to seek psychiatric help.

Sarcasm expressed as a statement or a question is meant to hurt, so it is difficult to think of an example to illustrate asking the question about religion. However, suppose a very insecure young man has been putting on a show of arrogance and insolence, then the question on religion might be phrased 'I don't suppose anyone as high and mighty as you needs religion, but I have to ask?' Sometimes it is the tone of voice rather than the actual question that implies sarcasm. Indeed it is important to remember that the tone and all other non-verbal cues, as well as the phrasing used when questioning, makes a lot of difference in establishing the trust that leads to thoughtful and meaningful information being shared even when it might be about embarrassing or threatening things.

Because mentally ill patients often experience difficulty in communicating spontaneously and because psychiatric nurses sometimes have to explore painful or embarrassing topics, it is essential they become skilled at eliciting information that is comprehensive, unbiased, and true for the patient and that they use their observation skills to gain information from both verbal and non-verbal responses to questions. As with observation skills, the way to improving questioning skills lies in increasing self-awareness and also in being prepared to listen to colleagues' constructive criticism.

(3) Listening Skills

The ability to listen actively and attentively is natural and easy when the speaker appeals to us and is interesting. What is difficult is being interested and appearing interested when the other person is uncommunicative, boringly repetitive or evasive.

Active listening requires a conscious effort to register and remember what is being said and then, later on, referring accurately to items that have been remembered. This provides one of our most potent tools for communicating that someone is 'worth' something to us.

It is a repeated criticism of the Nursing Process that patients on admission are asked their wishes in various respects and then no attention is paid to them. If this does occur it has the negative effect of making the patient feel more ignored or rejected than if he had not been asked in the first place and can lead to feelings of helplessness and anger. From this point of view it is important not to fall into the trap of asking questions and listening only to what we want to hear when filling in an assessment document. Apart from data for the face sheet of the document, it is probably better to make brief notes of the assessment interview and transfer them to the document later. Beginners need broad headings to remind them what to notice and where to direct enquiry, but the patient is more likely to feel at ease if he is not being 'quizzed'.

For on-going assessment it is important to listen for the moment when something stops being a problem or when the patient changes his viewpoint. There are definitely times when we hope others will actively forget something about us or something we have said, but this can only be found out with ongoing listening and feedback of new rememberings.

Listening in order to collect information, as with observation and questioning, is a learned skill. The ability to use non-verbal cues to communicate interest, to make silence comfortable, to make embarrassing disclosures safe or to stem the flow of a tirade that has become repetitive, are skills many psychiatric nurses possess. Nevertheless they can with awareness and practice usually be improved.

(4) Recording Skills

Recording the assessment of a patient falls into two main parts. There is the information that is needed for administrative and legal requirements. This is referred to as 'face sheet' or 'front sheet' data and will be familiar to all nurses. There should be a standard format for this sheet, but whether the standard applies to a Unit, a hospital, a district or even nationally will depend on management policy. Chapter 8 on documentation gives some examples of 'face sheets' but for now it will suffice to say that the information on the face sheet identifies the patient and the relatively unchanging facts about him.

The other elements of an assessment pose several problems when it comes to recording them. Once a form has been designed, it should be easy to fill in. However, it is in the nature of an assessment of a mentally ill person that the amount of information which is needed to be gained can be extensive. The first skill therefore has to be to decide what to put in and what to leave out and the document will influence this to a considerable extent.

As well as influencing how much information can be recorded, the document may well influence what type of information is recorded. For example, a psychogeriatric ward may include a base line daily living skills assessment chart, while an acute ward might include a social interaction inventory, or they might provide

Figure 3.1: Summarising Assessment Chart Based on the Psychiatric Nursing Grid (Normally set as an A4 chart)

Shade in outer band of segment for dependency level of care.
Shade in middle band of segment for supervisory level of care.
Shade in inner band of segment for independence.

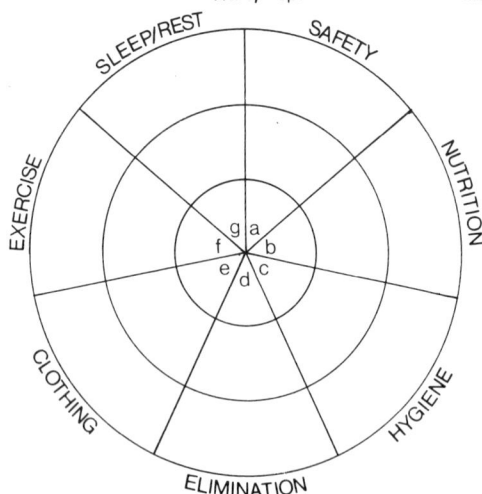

Physical Aspects
a. safety; b; nutrition; c. hygiene; d. elimination; e. clothing; f. exercise/mobility; g. sleep/rest

Figure 3.1 — *continued*

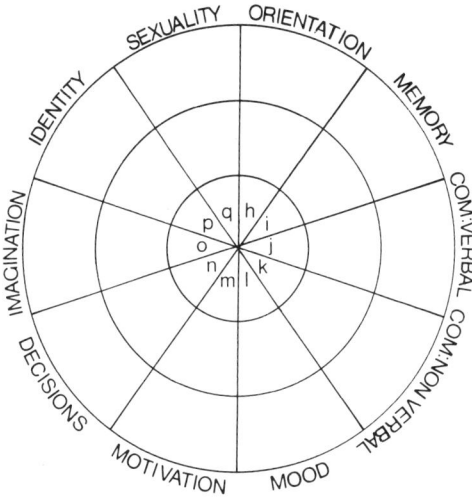

Psychological Aspects
h. orientation; i. memory; j. communication — verbal; k. communication — non-verbal; l. mood; m. motivation; n. decision-making; o. imagination/creativity; p. identity (ego strength); q. sexuality

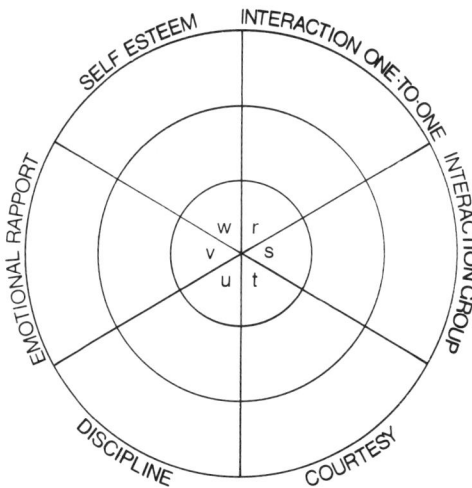

Social Aspects
r. interaction — one-to-one; s. interaction — group; t. courtesy/consideration; u. discipline/obedience; v. emotional rapport; w. self-esteem/self-confidence

just a blank piece of paper or card or a few generalised headings. Yet, whatever the form of the document or any supplementary charts that are decided upon, there are some skills in recording information that will ensure a better foundation on which to build a plan of care.

The first thing is to ensure that facts rather than the nurse's value judgements are recorded, or that any such value judgements are made explicit. For example, to describe someone on admission as being disturbed and unco-operative conveys very little information about him, but the words will evoke feelings and preconceptions in other readers. Such readers may experience these as fact and may well be influenced in their approach to, and interaction with, the patient.

The behaviour that was described as 'disturbed and un-co-operative' could have been more helpfully recorded, for example, as 'Repeatedly stood up to look in drawers and leave the room while being interviewed. Did not respond to his name, but sat for a few minutes when directed. Mute, so far, when questioned but nods or shakes head. Has spoken once when asking for a drink shortly after refusing his tea.'

There is no denying that recording facts accurately takes more effort, time and space, but practice makes it easier to pinpoint incidents that can communicate a lot of information. Whatever the format of the documents when the assessment is completed, there should be a factual outline 'profile' of the patient that gives a physical description and highlights any areas where there is a threat to safety, the main nursing needs or problems, major likes or dislikes and particular strengths and abilities. An assessment summary needs to be available for speedy reference, but also for newcomers to the nursing team. This profile, like the rest of the assessment information, needs to be recorded in such a way that it is possible to make changes or additions as the patient becomes better known or his condition changes. It is important to recognise that a documented assessment is not sacrosanct and if contradictory facts are noticed they should find room to be recorded.

In acute wards the initial assessment will probably serve the patient's stay in hospital, but in long-stay areas it is important to re-assess patients at least once a year. Ideally this re-assessment should be done by someone who does not know the patient very well and should be done without reference to the previous records. This may sound time-consuming, but it can be an on-going exercise throughout the year, as it can when a ward first changes to using the Nursing Process approach to nursing care.

Mention has been made of charts that have been devised for recording different aspects of a patient's behaviour. There are several of these and they can be useful for summarising observations, especially where rapid changes are expected. They can serve as a useful adjunct to a good nursing assessment, but must not be filled in from guesswork just for the sake of completing the form.

Figure 3.1 shows an assessment chart that is based on the psychiatric nursing grid discussed in Chapter 5 (p. 42). Wherever the outer circle is shaded one would expect to see details of a relevant nursing intervention in the care plan.

If any aspect of the patient's care needs particular attention, then that area of the circle can be shaded in a different colour. For example, a patient who aggravates his fellows with taunting and sarcasm would have the outer circle of the 'group interaction' highlighted, or a depressed suicidal patient would have the 'safety' and 'mood' outer circles highlighted. Such charts can be updated as necessary or at prescribed time intervals.

Another useful acivity that can help give a more complete picture of a particular aspect of a patient's behaviour, is recording observations on a time-sampling basis. Such 'base-line' observations can complement an assessment profile, but like assessment charts must be an additional exercise.

Summary

The assessment of a patient produces a written account of information, gained from as many sources as possible, that is factual, accurate and relevant. It should provide an individualised picture of the patient, his strengths and difficulties, his likes and dislikes, so that the team has a sound basis for deciding what nursing will be most helpful.

4 PLANNING: AGREEING WHAT NURSING NEEDS DOING

The purpose of making plans is to organise the future in order to achieve some objective. Plans should be possible to carry out and not just paper exercises or castles in the air, and they should allow for flexibility if circumstances change.

In the interests of the Nursing Process a nursing care plan must be based on the accurate assessment of the patient and be set towards realistic objectives. In our less than ideal world it must identify the essential priorities for each patient as there are unlikely to be enough nurses or time to provide ideal care for everyone. All members of the nursing team should contribute to the drawing up of a plan of care but there will always be times when an individual nurse has to make a decision about an immediate action in the interests of the patient's safety or because circumstances indicate that an agreed plan is not still relevant.

Wherever possible it is useful to encourage the patient to participate in deciding what nursing care is likely to prove most beneficial. Quite often the patient does know best what may be helpful to him, but even if his ideas are not realistic, it is usually possible to plan some aspect of care with him in which he can actively play some part and feel he has some autonomy and responsibility.

Knowledge Needed for Planning Nursing Care

(1) Enough knowledge of the theory and practice of nursing to know what is likely to be effective, safe and possible to carry out.
(2) A knowledge of the law as it relates to professional accountability, the duty of caring and justifiable risk.

Skills Needed for Planning Nursing Care

(1) The ability to identify and state objectives or goals.

(2) The ability to make conscious and put into words the whole range of nursing skills and interventions.
(3) The ability to predict the best choice of nursing interventions to reach a specified objective.
(4) The ability to establish priorities as to what nursing care is most important for each individual patient, and as to which patients are most in need of the skills and the time available.
(5) The ability to decide the best choice of nursing intervention.
(6) The ability to summarise and write down agreed plans.

(1) The Ability to Identify and State Objectives

When members of the nursing team have got to know the patient they are in a position to decide what nursing he needs. It is one of the many disciplines of the Nursing Process to be able to identify and state clear goals or objectives. These two terms are interchangeable, but practice is coming to identify objectives with short-term targets (tactical planning) and goals with more long-term ones (strategic planning).

Some writers refer to 'behavioural objectives'. These are very specific and it is easy to identify whether the nursing provided has achieved the objective. A behavioural objective is stated in such terms as 'Mr Jones will be able to go to the shops on his own initiative and purchase what he wants by (date).' Because such objectives are so very specific it is useful to be able to express patients' nursing needs in such terms, but in psychiatric nursing practice comprehensive objectives may be more useful because the nature of the care required is so complex. The above example might be included in an objective that is stated as 'to increase his independence'. There can be a danger if objectives are stated in terms that are too vague because there will be too many alternative interventions to choose from and it will prove very difficult to decide if the objective has been achieved. An example of a vague objective would be 'improve social skills' and a vague goal would be 'rehabilitation'.

(2) Putting Nursing Skills and Interventions into Words

In practice it is probably easier to put the physical aspects of psychiatric nursing into words than the psychological ones. It is easy to write 'Toilet two-hourly and chart' for the lady described in Chapter 2, although plans that seem straightforward can be interpreted by different people in different ways. The 'two-hourly toileting' can be understood as: (i) reminding the patient and putting a tick on a chart for the reminder; (ii) directing the patient to the toilet door, seeing her enter and ticking as a result of that; or (iii) ensuring she goes into the toilet and finding out whether she made use of the visit and charting that. The next chapter explains about writing nursing orders or instructions that translate the care plan into action and it is even more important that these should convey the same meaning for everyone concerned.

At the present time it is quite difficult to find plans of nursing care in psychiatric wards. What there is, is usually found in the report book or Kardex® with an observation such as 'Very withdrawn today. Encourage socialisation' for one patient and 'Still full of complaints and reluctant to eat. All tests N.A.D. Reassure', for another. Nursing Care Plans need more specific wording and this means that nurses need to know what particular action does encourage socialisation or what intervention might be reassuring.

A planning discussion about these patients might lead to a decision that the withdrawn person should be able to manage the dining room but not the ward meeting or other social activities. The plan would then state for the short term 'Meals in dining room. May sit on own, but not lie on bed. One-to-one interaction as appropriate — observe eye contact and verbal responses.'

An underlying component aim of all psychiatric nursing is to ensure that the patient's needs for self-esteem and individuality are met. Most nurses have found their own techniques for doing this, but there is only a narrow margin between making someone feel good or making him feel belittled and patronised. Because of this it is very difficult to find the words to put this aspect of nursing into a care plan.

The planning discussion for the second quoted example might lead the team to a decision that this patient needed to be helped to feel welcome in the ward even though she denies any psychiatric problems and no physical cause has been found for her symptoms. It may decide that gaining an understanding of the part anxiety may be playing and relaxation tuition might be useful and that she needed to be helped to feel likeable by staff and other patients — or in other words, her psychological needs must be met.

At this point the reader should try and write down a plan of nursing care to meet these objectives . . .

How well have you managed?

This example has been chosen because of the very real difficulty of translating 'ensure psychological needs are met' into specific nursing terms. A partial solution lies in recognising that what makes people feel good is being sought out for their company and having things remembered about them, such as what they have said, or what has been noticed. With that in mind a care plan could indicate that 'unsolicited' or 'unasked' time be given to the patient by one, some or all of the team members and the duration of the time could also be specified.

There is a suggested nursing care plan for the second patient in Appendix 4 and it is placed there so you can make your own attempt before referring to it.

(3) The Ability to Predict and Decide Upon the Best Nursing Intervention

When a patient has what seems an intractable problem, nurses are often heard to say 'we have tried everything' and although they may be hard put to say what the 'everything' has been, the phrase does indicate that often there are choices of nursing intervention. It takes experience to decide which might be the most helpful strategy at a particular time. However, it takes the discipline of the nursing process philosophy to ensure that the choice of action, having been agreed, is carried out by all members of the team, and for long enough to evaluate its effectiveness.

The ability to foresee and forestall problems also comes with experience. The nurse needs to take an active interest in patients to store information about them so that it is retrievable when circumstances require it. For this reason good, well recorded, assessments can provide valuable pointers for decision-making.

For example, an elderly patient, when being re-assessed, might have been found to have a rather low blood pressure. Later, when she shows an unusual reluctance to get out of bed in the mornings a check of her blood pressure for postural hypotension and particular observation of giddiness would lead to the care plan stating 'support when rising from bed or chair; supervise in the toilet; record lying and standing B/P daily a.m.' and this would be reported to the medical staff. In psychiatric nursing there is quite a chance that even if postural hypotension is found, it may well be nothing to do with, or only part of, the reason for this patient not getting up in the morning. In this case it could perhaps be that this lady is grieving for a friend in the ward who has recently died or maybe it is a depressive phase of a long term cyclical illness. In such a case cossetting her and allowing her to 'lie in' if she wishes might be more appropriate care. The point to be made is that the better the knowledge about the patient and the present circumstances, the more likely is the chosen nursing intervention to be a helpful one.

(4) Establishing Priorities of Nursing Care

Many nurses feel that the Nursing Process involves a lot of writing and this would be true if everything every patient needed from the nursing team was written down. In any ward there will be a 'baseline' or communal aspect of nursing provision that applies to all patients and it is only different or additional nursing care that needs to be recorded.

The first priority of nursing care has to be the patients' safety and their physical well-being. If these aspects are catered for by the basic provision in the ward then the next priority will be the management of whatever is proving to be most distressing for the patient, whether this be psychological or physical distress. Eventually the priority for nursing care will be whatever most helps the patient towards independence, contentment and recovery, or to feel comfortably 'at home' where recovery is not possible. In deciding what aspect of nursing care is most important for an individual patient, the short-term objectives will need most consideration. Yet it is still important to bear the long-term goals in mind and to see the overall nursing care as a series of planned sequences.

Another factor that influences decisions about what nursing it is important to do first, is relating the amount of nursing time and skill available to the nursing needs of all the patients, and ensuring that the nursing care is shared safely and fairly between them all. It is this factor that in many instances limits the number of objectives that can realistically be put into the short-term stage of a nursing care plan.

(5) Deciding the Best Choice of Nursing Intervention

This ability requires a sound knowledge of nursing practice, but it is helped towards its achievement by a clear statement of the objectives that are being worked towards, and by a sharing of the decision-making process. Quite often when trying to agree on a nursing strategy it is realised that more information is needed, so the first nursing objective would be 'To gain factual information about . . .' and the nursing action 'Observe and record all incidents of . . . and any precipitating factors.' At the review date it is possible that there might be a lead to a decision about the best course of action.

There are several broad categories of intervention when the nursing team is faced with problem behaviour:

(a) to accept it;
(b) to ignore it;
(c) to use rewards;
(d) to use 'punishments';
(e) to use distraction;
(f) to offer alternatives;
(g) to anticipate and prevent the need to manifest the problem behaviour.

Nurses probably use some sort of check list like this at an unconscious level, but in shared planning and decision-making, it is useful to have such a list available to work through together.

Arriving at a shared decision about the best nursing intervention means that nurses must be able to justify to their colleagues why they think one course of action would be better than another. This is an ability that becomes easier with practice and is another of the benefits of using the Nursing Process. When a decision about the main nursing strategy has been agreed then decisions about how best to implement it should be easier.

As previously stated nurses are sometimes heard to say 'we have tried everything' when faced with intractably difficult behaviour in psychiatric patients. With the discipline of the Nursing Process there will be a record of the 'everything' and an indication as to which of the different strategies were most or least helpful. There will also be the knowledge that the same strategy was being used by all the nurses for the stated period of time.

(6) Summarising and Writing Down Agreed Plans

Where the assessment of the patient has been recorded accurately and competently, it should lead the nurse to an expectation of what nursing decisions should have been or should be made. What is written down in a care plan will depend mainly on two factors: First, the type of nursing record used and how much space is available and secondly, the model of nursing on which practice is based. Headings for the nursing care plan sheet are discussed in Chapter 8 on documentation, but whichever headings are used it is important that what is written down is factual and specific. Generalisations are the biggest pitfall in all the stages of the Nursing Process, but it is in writing care plans and nursing orders that they should particularly be avoided.

An example of a generalised nursing instruction would be 'encourage good social skills'. With good assessment the team should know whether it was the patient's manners that were unacceptable or his difficulty in being with people, or in making conversation, or all of these that needed help. As has been stated, the choice of nursing intervention is wide but some examples of specific nursing plans could be 'Draw his attention to incidents when manners are unacceptable and suggest or model suitable alternatives, N.B. meal times'; 'Introductions and interactions with other patients — one or two per day'; 'To join recreational activities — give acknowledgement and praise for any participation'.

Whatever Nursing Process documentation is in use and on whatever basis the nursing care is being planned, it is likely that there will be a limit to the amount of space available for writing down the plan. One solution is to use abbreviations and this is permissible providing they are meaningful to all the staff and to any newcomers.

Another factor that helps to shorten care plans is the recognition that in all wards there is a 'common denominator' of nursing provision that is given to all patients. This should be recorded as 'ward policy' and will refer to such things as the patients' freedom to leave the ward, access to the kitchen, attendance at ward meetings, daily programmes of activities, etc. In any aspect where the agreed plan of nursing care falls within this 'shared' provision, it will not need to be recorded for an individual patient. It is only where the generalised care does not apply or something more specific is needed that it has to be written down on the care plan and then, as stated when discussing decisions about priorities of nursing care, only three or four items should be on the plan at any one time.

Summary

Nursing care plans are an agreed written account of the specific nursing care that it is felt will help the patient towards the objectives identified from the nursing assessment. They should communicate, in unambiguous language, what nursing care the patient needs, and which aspects are most important for both the short-term objectives and the longer-term goals. Agreeing the content of the plans should be a team activity, and where possible the patient should be encouraged to participate in reaching the decisions.

5 NURSING ORDERS: INSTRUCTING WHO DOES WHAT NURSING, FOR WHOM, AND WHEN

Making a plan is just a theoretical exercise until it is translated into action. Nursing orders are the instructions given to nurses to translate the plan into actual nursing. Sometimes nursing instructions are explicit from the written plan and where individual patients are allocated to a particular nurse there might be no need for further direction. One such example is given in Section 2(b) of the care plan in Appendix 4, where it is evident that no further instruction is needed for a designated nurse to know what to do.

However, some nursing may have been planned to be carried out only in a particular circumstance and the nurses need to know whether that circumstance applies. Likewise, some nursing is planned to be given weekly or, maybe, as often as possible and the nurses need to know who is to carry out the planned care on any particular shift. For example, a patient might be assessed as being actively suicidal. The objective could state 'To prevent self-harm'; the nursing action might state 'Nurse in bed with constant observation' or 'Special in bed' or 'Bed care with 1 : 1 nursing'. Whichever way it is expressed the plan indicates that a nurse must be with the patient all the time, but should it be one nurse all day, being relieved for meal breaks, should it be two nurses alternating, or should all the nurses take an hour each? The choice will depend on many factors but a decision has to be made and the nurses need to know.

As stated previously, the Nursing Process is sometimes described as an individualised approach to nursing care and this can be interpreted as meaning that individual members of the nursing team should care for individual or small groups of patients. Small teams of nurses caring for larger groups of specified patients is sometimes seen as an alternative. Community psychiatric nursing has to be organised on a patient assignment system, but faced with the reality of the staffing of psychiatric wards, with limited or fluctuating numbers and changing mixes of qualified staff, learners and nursing assistants, there is the possibility that sharing the nursing workload on a 'task assignment' basis may be the only possible strategy for deploying the available 'pairs of hands'. Although different nurses doing different tasks for the patient can tend to 'disintegrate' and distance them, this is probably more true in general wards than psychiatric ones, where patients are likely to stay longer and all the nurses get to know them as individuals to some degree at least.

There is no doubt that if the activities of assessing, planning and deciding who does what nursing are discussed and shared, there can be enough individualising of the patients and their needs to satisfy the Nursing Process philosophy. When it is decided which nurses are to do what nursing then the particular nursing activities have to be clearly specified.

For the example above, 'specialing', 'constant observation' and 'one-to-one nursing' can all indicate the same nursing care, but each can also have different meanings at different times and in different places. Can the patient go into the toilet on his own? Can the nurse leave while visitors are present? With regard to 'bed care', can the patient sit out for meals or go to the day room in a dressing gown if restless in bed?

It is in the 'doing of nursing' that nurses act most on intuition and unquestioned custom. Fortunately quite a lot of nursing is 'common sense' but in the realm of skilled nursing, for the safe care of the patient, for the training of learners and to ensure legal and professional responsibility, it is essential to be specific and to be able to write down detailed nursing instructions.

With regard to the Nursing Process it may be impossible to be so detailed on each patient's record, but already in some wards there are such things as written procedures or instructions for 'anorexia nervosa regime' or 'modified insulin care' or 'pre- and post-ECT care'. If the most commonly used nursing interventions were detailed in a ward 'nursing activities book' then only deviations from the standard pattern need be written on the patient's record. Thus there might be three levels of 'specialising' detailed, with level one setting the requirements for care where it is essential that the patient is observed at all times, and level three perhaps setting down what 'keeping an eye on' involved, when the patient is better and more trust has been gained. Level two would detail the stage in between.

As implementing the Nursing Process is essentially a team activity, it is important that detailing the relevant nursing activities must be a group effort and must be modified in the light of experience and as times change and new knowledge is gained.

Whether each ward would have to draw up its own 'nursing activities book' or whether wards with similar groups of patients could co-operate, or even if it would be possible for a psychiatric division to arrive at standardised nursing actions, is a point for consideration.

However they are arrived at, it is important to remember that written 'nursing actions' recorded for general application must not become rigid routines. Their prime purpose is to ensure that there is agreement between nurses as to what nursing they are expected to do in any particular circumstance, but they must always be related to each individual patient with a view to deciding whether any aspects do not apply or whether anything needs to be added or modified. In these circumstances it is only these deviations from the standard pattern that would be recorded on the patient's nursing record.

The following suggests a sample 'nursing activity' entry for reality orientation in psychogeriatric assessment ward. For this exercise reality orientation is the ongoing nursing interaction rather than a formal Reality Orientation session.

Reality Orientation — Continuous. Record as 24 hr r.o.

During interaction with the patient, while attending to activities of daily living, and during recreactional activities, where natural and as frequently as possible:

(1) Use the patient's name (see preferred name on Kardex).
(2) Indicate time of day, day of week, time of year and where they are.
(3) Encourage patient to identify own bed,
own chair,
own clothes,
own possessions,
your name/role.
(4) Give the opportunity to find his own way around the ward, but direct tactfully if he cannot do it.
(5) Speak only when the patient can see you and give time for a reply.
(6) Ensure 'memory aids' in the ward are up to date and accurate (e.g. a teddy on the bed must be the right teddy

and the daily paper must be today's).

(7) Draw the patient's attention to 'memory' and 'reality' through such things as TV, food, weather, visitors, etc.

(8) Give a few minutes' warning of the next activity, e.g. toileting, meals and bedtime.

(9) Listen to reminiscences and try and relate them to the present.

(10) Always give the patient the opportunity to use his memory but help him out before he experiences distress.

This example of a recorded nursing activity is not offered as a definitive description of reality orientation, but is included to show that however much the reader might agree or disagree, it took less than half an hour to jot down. Having said this, it is important to remember that an individual producing her own ideas is not what the Nursing Process philosophy is about. This example should be left where it belongs — in the pages of this book — while individuals as members of ward teams decide what they mean by 'reality orientation' as a nursing intervention in their particular ward.

As nursing teams discipline themselves to record their nursing activities and then achieve this, so they become more aware of what nursing they are doing and should continuously make additions and alterations to the nursing activity records as habit. With a 'nursing activites book' containing an entry for reality orientation it would be sufficient to enter on a newly admitted patient's record, '24 hr r.o. — all nurses'. If it happened that this was a severely demented patient who became extremely agitated at any suggestion that she was in hospital then the entry could read '24 hr r.o. — all nurses, but collude with her belief that she is in a hotel'.

If all the patients in a ward are severely demented then continuing reality orientation would be part of the communal basic provision and would be included in the ward nursing policy document and would not have to be referred to on each patient's record.

Because it is difficult to isolate specific nursing actions from the overall activity of nursing, the grid in Table 5.1 is presented to help focus on discreet aspects of the patients' behaviour. Thus nursing interventions appropriate for the patient's age, illness and prognosis can be agreed upon for each item. This grid encourages nurses to look at their nursing as on a continuum, with the patient being entirely dependent on them at one end of the scale, to being

Table 5.1: Aspects of Psychiatric Nursing for Care Plans and Nursing Actions

	Physical Aspects	Psychological Aspects	Social Aspects
Independence Care	a. Safety b. Nutrition c. Hygiene d. Elimination e. Clothing f. Exercise/Mobility g. Sleep/Rest	h. Orientation i. Memory j. Communication — verbal k. Communication — non-verbal l. Mood m. Motivation n. Decision-making o. Imagination/Creativity p. Identity (Ego strength) q. Sexuality	r. Interaction — one-to-one s. Interaction — group t. Courtesy/Consideration u. Discipline/Obedience v. Emotional rapport w. Self-esteem/Confidence
Supervisory Care	a. Safety b. Nutrition c. Hygiene d. Elimination e. Clothing f. Exercise/Mobility g. Sleep/Rest	h. Orientation i. Memory j. Communication — verbal k. Communication — non-verbal l. Mood m. Motivation n. Decision-making o. Imagination/Creativity p. Identity (Ego strength) q. Sexuality	r. Interaction — one-to-one s. Interaction — group t. Courtesy/Consideration u. Discipline/Obedience v. Emotional rapport w. Self-esteem/Confidence
Dependence Care	a. Safety b. Nutrition c. Hygiene d. Elimination e. Clothing f. Exercise/Mobility g. Sleep/Rest	h. Orientation i. Memory j. Communication — verbal k. Communication — non-verbal l. Mood m. Motivation n. Decision-making o. Imagination/Creativity p. Identity (Ego strength) q. Sexuality	r. Interaction — one-to-one s. Interaction — group t. Courtesy/Consideration u. Discipline/Obedience v. Emotional rapport w. Self-esteem/Confidence

able to manage on their own at the other, and needing supervision and help in between. It should also help nurses to see that any particular patient may be independent in some respects, but need supervision or dependency care in others.

Another way in which such a grid can prove helpful is in directing the nurse's attention towards both short-term and longer-term objectives. The nursing actions that are considered to be best for the moment are prescribed and in addition a start can be made on decisions about longer-term strategies. An example of this might be the nursing orders for a patient whose every penny and every waking moment is devoted to getting and smoking cigarettes. The short-term objective might be to reduce his smoking to twenty cigarettes a day by a specified date, while the long-term objective would be for him to have self-control over his money and his smoking. The initial nursing orders could state:

(1) Hand out ten cigarettes at 9.00 a.m. and 2.00 p.m. Staff to control and supervise any spending money.
(2) Encourage attendance at programmed activities. Observe smoking behaviour and provide distraction and discouragement.
(3) Key worker to engage interest and discuss saving money for some item of his choice.

Item (1) is a nursing order for the dependency level of care. Item (2) is an instruction to all nurses at a supervisory level of care, while item (3) is the first stage of the key worker's role in implementing a plan for the long-term goal.

This shows how it is possible for a team to be working at various levels even when managing a specific difficulty.

The actual items in the grid are, as with other things in this book, only offered as a starting point for discussion, but it is probably necessary to have some overview when thinking about and writing specific nursing instructions. Referring to the example grid for the time being, the account of reality orientation detailed above would correspond to dependency care for orientation in a psychogeriatric ward, but would need to be modified if applied to a very hallucinated youngster in an acute admission ward.

Likewise, in a psychogeriatric ward, dependency care for nutrition will probably entail actually feeding the patient. An independent patient will manage to eat on her own, so the independency care would be to ensure appetising food is served and other patients do not interfere. In an acute ward, dependency care for nutrition might be needed for someone with severe depression or anorexia nervosa, while independency care would concentrate on ensuring a good social atmosphere in the dining room. Whether such patients are served or help themselves should be a ward nursing policy decision and, like everything else, discussed and recorded.

If these examples make the task of compiling a nursing activities book seem too formidable, it should be evident that for any particular ward the major part of nursing care will fall within one or two 'boxes' of the grid. If the most appropriate aspects are tackled first then the others can be done later as it, hopefully, gets easier.

Summary

Nursing orders, sometimes referred to as nursing prescriptions, are specific written instructions that translate the nursing care plan into action.

If shorthand terms or abbreviations are used on the patient's record, the full instructions should nevertheless be available. It is suggested that specific psychiatric nursing interventions could be recorded in a book so that entries can be brief, but will refer to an agreed strategy. Then only deviations or additions to the agreed strategy need be written on an individual patient's record. Nursing orders, besides indicating what nursing is to be carried out, must identify who is to do what nursing, when and how often.

6 IMPLEMENTATION: DOING THE NURSING

Doing the nursing is the most important part of the Nursing Process and yet this chapter is one of the shortest in the book. This reflects the problem that some people have experienced in undertaking to implement the Nursing Process. They feel that the assessment, planning and documentation takes so much time that there is less time available for actually caring for patients.

The foregoing chapters have indicated that it does indeed take time to practise and become skilled at recording useful, factual profiles and assessments of patients; it will need time to verbalise and record relevant nursing actions; it will take time to develop and learn to use appropriate documentation. This however, has to be regarded as 'invested' time, because, once the skills are mastered, nursing actions are in conscious awareness and recorded and the documentation is satisfactory, then the time spent on discussion and writing should get less and the time available for nursing intervention increase. The benefit from this 'invested' time should be an increased awareness of what nursing each patient needs at any moment in time. It should also help the nursing team to be aware of choices of nursing intervention, to agree on the best choice and enable it to justify any particular decision. Another benefit to the patients is that with well drawn-up nursing care plans there should be more equitable sharing of nursing teams' time and skills than is often the case at the present time. As this is not a textbook of psychiatric nursing there is no place here for an account of 'doing the nursing', but there are some aspects of implementing the nursing that need some mention.

It is perhaps timely to recall our definition of the Nursing Process. It is a *systematic* way of: *consciously* thinking about patients; ensuring that what *each* patient needs is *identified*; organising and doing the nursing; checking and *recording* that the required nursing has been carried out, and *evaluating* the effectiveness of the care given.

There is nothing in that definition, or in the foregoing chapters, that puts into words a very important aspect of any caring activity, in that, it is not so much *what* is done but *how* it is done that is important in influencing standards of care. Each of the emphasised words in the definition has relevance to implementing the planned nursing as well as embodying the philosophy of the Nursing Process. Being systematic while doing the nursing means organising the work efficiently and making maximum use of the available resources, but it also means basing practice on sound factual knowledge and being accountable for the care that is carried out.

Accountability is being able to accept personal responsibility for the nursing one has done, being able to justify the choice of intervention and the way in which it was carried out. This can only be done when nursing practice is based on sound knowledge and fact, rather than on intuition and hunch.

Because psychiatric nursing, in quite large part, involves using interpersonal skills to help patients, it is tempting to go along with the idea that good psychiatric nurses 'are born, and not made'. However, there are some research reports, listed at the end of this chapter, which indicate that what nurses are thought to do, what they think they do and what they actually do, is at some variance. There are some aspects of these interpersonal skills that need to be brought to conscious awareness for this aspect of nursing to be objectively based, so that individual nurses can be accountable for the interpersonal aspects of their care.

Nursing textbooks lay emphasis on the importance of the relationship between nurse and patient, of gaining trust and guiding, counselling, exploring, motivating and otherwise making the relationship 'therapeutic'. These are useful and necessary skills, but the research projects referred to above indicate that not very much nursing time is spent at that level of interaction. Instead nurses are observed to do quite a lot of chatting and patients have expressed that they enjoy and are helped by nurses who can chat about everday things in a friendly manner.

Experience suggests that there is a limit to the amount of 'therapeutic' interaction that any individual can tolerate. There are some patients for whom 'in-depth' intervention from nurses is not appropriate, so the ability to help patients feel noticed and likeable through friendly chat possibly plays a considerable part in generating a therapeutic environment.

This point about conversation can be used to illustrate the fact that it is not so much what is done but how it is done that is important in implementing nursing. Because chatting is so normal and nurses are human it is easy for them to behave as normal and chat to people who are responsive and on the same wavelength. However, many people who are mentally ill have difficulty in initiating or maintaining social chit-chat, so it is likely to be those who are least incapacitated or furthest on the way to recovery with whom the nurses choose to chat during any slack moments in the day or while they are carrying out nursing activities for them. Meanwhile, patients less able to participate are left feeling out of things and comparatively deprived.

If this aspect of nursing interaction is recognised by the team as being important and allowable, it can then be prescribed in nursing orders and its effect evaluated for all patients. It must be done in an aware, yet natural manner for it to be a beneficially skilled intervention. It is possible that a nurse may chat in a very self-centred way that does not allow or encourage any response or involvement and this can be potentially harmful, while a small group chatting in a way that excludes others can be equally detrimental.

There is another aspect of psychiatric nursing where *how* the nursing is done is of paramount importance. Most nurses will have sensed, although not necessarily been aware, that sometimes patients seem to be very well cared for even though nothing much is going on at the time. Just because a particular nurse or team of nurses are on duty, their presence alone can reduce tension, allay anxiety or inspire motivation. This occurs because the nurses have gained the patients' confidence and trust by the manner in which they have carried out nursing activities previously.

Unfortunately, this aspect of care is impossible to prescribe because, conversely, it can happen that nurses may be doing harm to patients when they appear to be doing nothing. This will be because the manner in which they have carried out nursing care previously has lacked interest and enthusiasm or been carried out clumsily, leaving patients dispirited and distrustful.

Just as cross-infection can be an indicator of poor standards of nursing care in a general hospital, so boredom can be an indicator of poor nursing care in a psychiatric ward. It is relevant to recall Florence Nightingale's statement that 'the hospital should do the patient no harm'. While it is unlikely that patients will be physically hurt by nurses, there are some ways in which they can be psychologically hurt.

Sometimes nurses can be patronising toward patients, treating them in a condescending manner; sometimes they can be angered into teasing or sarcasm; sometimes they can be over-caring and protective, denying the patient individuality and autonomy and sometimes through lack of skill, resources or low morale, care is carried out in a mechanistic way that can leave the patients feeling bored and helpless. These things can happen, sometimes as an isolated incident or maybe for a particular patient, but occasionally as a regular pattern of the team's care.

If an agreed nursing care plan has been implemented and is found not to be effective, it is worth the team members exploring and examining their own and each other's attitudes and practice, in order to determine whether any of the negative aspects might be hindering recovery, rather than simply accepting that the chosen strategy was the wrong one.

The reference to *each* patient in the definition of the Nursing Process also has implications for doing the nursing. The philosophy of the Nursing Process requires that nurses get to know all their patients well and wherever possible involve them in planning their own care. This is fine when the patients are likeable and co-operative, but where patients make the nurse feel angry or helpless it is much more threatening to try to get closer. Isobel Menzies in 1960 suggested that in general nursing, the organisation of nursing work by assigning different tasks to different nurses was a means of providing emotional protection. In Chapter 5 on Nursing Orders it was suggested that organising work on a task assignment basis might be the only possibility in some wards, but this has to be on the assumption that all the nurses know all the patients well and are all involved in the care planning and carrying out the plans.

If the Nursing Process is going to be implemented successfully for all the patients in a ward, it is essential to identify individual and team antagonisms towards patients. For this to happen, the nurses have to feel safe enough with their colleagues to share very personal or negative feelings. This can only occur when the carers care for, and support, each other: recognising their own and others' strengths and limitations, sharing their skills and their feelings, their successes and failures, giving praise and criticism.

Nursing at the point of delivery is always a very personal activity but individualised nursing has to be teamwork. The stages and tools of the Nursing Process are entirely dependent on teamwork, but the whole investment of time, energy, skill and enthusiasm should ensure that the quality of nursing care given by each and every nurse be enhanced and beneficial.

Suggested Further Reading and References: Research Reports Relating to Psychiatric Nursing

Altschul, A. T. *Patient-Nurse Interaction* (Churchill Livingstone, Edinburgh, 1972)
Cormack, D. *Psychiatric Nursing Observed* (Royal College of Nursing, London, 1976)
—— *Psychiatric Nursing Described* (Churchill Livingstone, Edinburgh, 1983)
Menzies, I. E. P. 'A case study in the functioning of social systems as a defence against anxiety.' *Human Relations*, Vol. 13 (1960), pp. 95–121
Miller, A. F. 'Nursing Process and patient care.' *Nursing Times*, Occasional Paper, Vol. 80, No. 13 (1984), pp. 56–8
Norton, D., McLaren, R., and Exton-Smith, A. N. *An Investigation of Geriatric Nursing Problems in Hospital* (Churchill Livingstone, Edinburgh, 1962)
Paykel, E. S., and Griffith, J. H. *Community Psychiatric Nursing for Neurotic Patients* (Royal College of Nursing, London, 1983)
Towell, D. *Understanding Psychiatric Nursing* (Royal College of Nursing, London, 1975)

7 EVALUATION: DECIDING WHETHER NURSING CARE HAS BEEN EFFECTIVE

When a nursing team has defined objectives, identified problems or assessed needs that must be met and has decided what nursing should be carried out, it is logical to reflect on whether these decisions proved possible to implement and whether they have had a good or an adverse effect.

Nurses have always been required to report on their activities and the patients in their care, but these reports have tended to become very generalised and stereotyped. The Nursing Process, for the evaluation stage, as for other stages, imposes discipline on nursing practice. To write 'good day' or 'no change' may well be a true record, but it does not indicate that the patient has received any nursing attention and you may have to refer back a long way to find out what is 'good' for that patient, or from what state there has been no change.

The evaluation stage of the Nursing Process has two parts to it. There is the ongoing daily noticing and recording of the nursing that has been carried out and its effect on the patient and there is the periodic review of the nursing care plan by the nursing team to decide if and what amendments are needed. The factual recording of required or relevant observations of the patient, a record of what nursing has been carried out and an account of its effectiveness has come to be referred to as the nursing report. Because this is very similar to what has been done by nurses throughout their careers it is proving a difficult aspect to adapt to the requirements for the Nursing Process, which are that entries must be specific and factual or they are not worth the time and space they take to record.

Chapter 8 on documentation suggests using a number reference system for identifying planned items of nursing care and nursing orders. If such a system has been well designed, it is legitimate to enter the item number and just tick it and sign it when the nursing has been carried out. If any change in the patient's condition relating to the item has been noticed, a short factual statement should be added. Using a number reference system can save time and space, but whether or not such a system is used the nursing 'report' must refer specifically to the nursing orders.

It was stated in Chapter 4 on planning that where there is an agreed basic provision of nursing care that is given to all the patients, it can be taken for granted that this has been carried out and it does not need to be entered on each patient's record. When a patient is receiving a lot of nursing care or needs many or frequent observations to be recorded it may be necessary to use a special chart. Such a chart may be pinned up on a board, kept by the patient or placed with the patient's record, but it must be referred to in the nursing report daily. Where it has been possible for the patient to be involved in the planning of his care it must be remembered to obtain his viewpoint as to how effective the nursing interventions are proving and to record this.

Who actually makes the entries for the nursing report in the patient's record will depend on local policy. It has to be remembered that should anything go amiss, it is this part of the record that will provide evidence. It does not matter how comprehensive the care plan may be, it remains a plan until it is implemented, and the implementation remains 'not proven' unless it has been recorded.

Where patient or team assignment is possible, it seems sensible for the designated nurse or the team leader to make the entries. Where work is allocated by task assignment, it may be that the nurse who carries out a specified task for a patient writes and signs that specific entry. It may be that the person in charge of the ward fills in all the entries, relying on reported information. Whoever does fill in the entries, it must be remembered that they are statements of nursing carried out and if written by a learner or nursing assistant should be countersigned by a qualified nurse.

This ongoing recording of how the care plan has been implemented, and how effective it has been, is one aspect of evaluation. The other aspect might better be called 'reviewing' because it requires the nursing team to refer to the care plan at regular intervals to decide whether the planned nursing has been, is being or has not been effective. On the basis of this evaluation, a decision then has to be reached whether to continue as before or to make changes. It is this reviewing stage that makes the Nursing Process a cyclical system.

There should be target dates written into the care plan indicating when it is hoped a particular objective will be achieved. There will be daily reference to the care plan and amendments made as necessary, but it is important for the team to review not only the specific items of the plan but also the plan as a whole. This must be done in the context of the other patients in the ward and take into account not only changes in the patient, but also changes in the nursing team and the ward environment. When a review of a patient's care plan has been undertaken this must be recorded on the nursing report sheet with mention of the item numbers of particular plans that have been changed.

8 DOCUMENTATION: PUTTING THE OTHER STAGES IN WRITING FOR COMMUNICATION AND REFERENCE

The foregoing chapters have described the stages of the Nursing Process and the adjustments that need to be made to current nursing practice for it to be implemented in psychiatric nursing. Throughout the book reference has been made to the necessity of recording the decisions reached and the actions taken. For the Nursing Process approach to function effectively, with nursing taking the priority in time and effort, the documentation must serve the team as a tool and not become a time-consuming burden. As with the other stages the time spent in planning and discussing alternative systems and the design of documents should prove a beneficial investment.

The means by which nursing assessments, plans, orders, reports and evaluations are recorded for keeping and sharing are, so far, on written forms. Computerised records may not be so far away but they will still need the same discipline of being accurate, concise and accessible.

Nurses are faced with deciding between two main types of written recording systems. These are sheets of paper held in a folder of some sort or cards in a holder. Before reaching a decision on which to use, nurses should be aware of the advantages and dis-advantages of each system and discuss the alternatives with the con-sultants and medical records officer as nursing 'reports' are restricted documents and as such will need to be stored after the patient's discharge or death (HM(61)73).

There are factors in favour of and factors against both systems and it could be that a folder system would suit community nurses and acute wards, while a card system might be the ideal for psycho-geriatric wards. It is unlikely that a Unit or even a District Health Authority would opt for using two different systems, so the one chosen should suit the majority. A review of the purpose that the nursing record must serve, together with the requirements imposed by adopting the Nursing Process concept should clarify the points that will influence a decision.

The first essential feature of the nursing documentation is to be able to identify the patient and relate the nursing record to the medical 'notes'. This information is sometimes referred to as 'face sheet' or 'front sheet' data and should contain the facts about the patient that are not likely to need amending very often. These face sheets will be familiar in some form to all nurses, but an example is given in Figure 8.1 to show that for some of the items it is possible to personalise some of the information to accord with the Nursing Process philosophy.

The second requirement is that the nursing record should provide enough space for what needs to be recorded, should have clear headings and where one part of the record refers to another part, both parts should be visible at the same time. The Nursing Process does dictate that there needs to be more sheets for the documentation than for a conventional nursing record, because it is impossible to fit the care plan, nursing orders, report and evaluation all on one page.

The final requirement is that the documentation should be manageable over a period of time. It has to be robust enough to undergo a lot of handling. It has to be tidy enough and secure enough to be stored or filed and yet be readily identified and accessible.

A Folder System for the Nursing Record

The first choice has to be what type of folder to use. There are envelope folders or flat folders, with or without holding mechanisms. The holding mechanisms can be springs in the spine of the folder, clip mechanisms or rings, or treasury tags to hold perforated pages. If at all possible these different systems should be observed in use to identify the benefits and shortcomings and the cost implications of each.

Having decided on the type of folder attention then has to be given to the sheets of paper, their size, the quality of the paper and possibly their colour. It might be decided to print the headings for the identification information (face sheet data) on the cover of the folder or perhaps use card for this sheet if it is going to have a lot of handling. If it is going to be held in place with rings or ties it is likely that the holes will need reinforcement. For the other documents it has been found helpful to use different coloured paper for the different forms to make it easy to identify what

Figure 8.1: Face Sheet Data

HEALTH AUTHORITY, PSYCHIATRIC UNIT

	Mr. Mrs. Miss M. S. W. SEP.	HOSPITAL/DEPT.	HOSPITAL No.
NAME		NAT. INS./PENSION NO.	
Likes to be called:		VALUABLES/MONEY IN HOSPITAL KEEPING YES/NO	
ADDRESS		HOSPITAL ACCOUNT NO.	
TEL. NO.		NEXT OF KIN:	
DATE OF BIRTH		— Relationship	
RELIGION		— Address	
RELIGIOUS PRACTICE			
OCCUPATION		— Tel. No.	
SOURCE OF REFERRAL		AND/OR SPECIAL FRIEND:	
		— Address	
GENERAL PRACTITIONER			
— Address			
		— Tel. No.	
— Tel. No.			
SOCIAL WORKER			
OTHER AGENCIES			

LEGAL STATUS	Expiry Date					
	Review Tribunal		GOOD	FAIR	POOR	AIDS	DATE CHECKED

		GOOD	FAIR	POOR	AIDS	DATE CHECKED
		SIGHT				
		HEARING				
DATE OF ADMISSION		SPEECH				
DATE OF TRANSFER	To:	TEETH				
DATE OF DISCHARGE		BALANCE				
— Follow-up		PROSTHESIS				
		ALLERGIES				

NAME	WARD/DEPT.	CONSULTANT

Figure 8.2: An Example of an Assessment Form

NAME   WARD   HOSPITAL NO.

HISTORY

ASSESSMENT

Physical state: Baseline Temp.   Pulse   Resp   B/P
Weight   Previous best weight
Urine
Date of last period (where relevant)
General description — re. general appearance, clothes, hygiene, posture, gait, etc.

Mental state: General description — re. attention, orientation, verbal and non-verbal skills, etc.

Emotional state: General description — re. expression, mood, etc.

Social skills/Relationships: Rapport, co-operation, friends, etc.

Patient's view of why he/she is needing care:

PROFILE

---

one is looking for in the folder.

The history, profile and assessment form can utilise the back of the face data sheet or it can be separate, but in either case is likely to need extra pages for keeping the assessment up-dated. Whether or not a separate sheet is used for this form the nature and number of headings will have to be agreed. For discussion about the alternatives the reader is referred to Chapter 3 on Assessment. One example is given here in Figure 8.2. Whatever format is decided upon there must be provision for recording changes in the patient's condition. Where an itemised list is used this will probably mean completing a new form at stated intervals or when necessary.

The assessment form can incorporate charts such as the Norton pressure sore risk scale, but it is probably better to enter the score on the observation record because when it is relevant it needs reassessing frequently, and the space on the assessment form can be more usefully used. An example of an assessment form is given in Figure 8.2.

The design of the sheets for nursing care plans will depend on the headings chosen and the number of columns needed. A4 size paper is most commonly available and this is rectangular in shape. This means the care plan can be set out with narrow but long columns or, if the paper is turned sideways, with wider but shorter columns. Whichever way is decided upon it is important that the rest of the nursing record documents are designed in the same orientation, because it makes it very difficult to use the folder if some sheets are printed lengthways and others sideways. Some example of headings for the Care Plan are given in Figure 8.3.

The documentation for recording the nursing orders and the observations, report and evaluation may fit on to one sheet or it may be better to use separate ones. Again, readers are referred to the relevant chapters and some suggested headings are given in Figures 8.4 and 8.5.

If different colours are used for the different forms of the nursing record, this makes it easier to find the current pages, especially if the last assessment entry on a sheet of one colour is placed next to the last care plan entry on a sheet of a different colour, and if the last nursing orders entry is placed adjacent to the last entry for report and evaluation, again with two different colours. This means the nurse only has to identify the two interface colour pages when using the folder, should the record become bulky when the patient has been in for some time. For this system

Figure 8.3: Examples of Headings for Nursing Care Plan Forms

Page.......

Date	Objectives	Nursing Plan	Review Date	Signature

Page.......

Date	Problems	Nursing Action	Review Date	Signature

Page.......

Date	Aims	Nursing Care Plan	Expected Outcome	Signature

Page.......

Date	Needs	Action	Sig.	Outcome	Sig.

Page.......

Date	Nursing Needs	Goals	Nursing Care	Evaluation

Figure 8.4: Examples of Headings for Nursing Orders Forms

Page.......

Date	Care Plan Ref. No.	Nursing Orders	Nurse Responsible	Signature

Page.......

Date	Care Plan Ref. No.	Nursing Action	Nurse	Time	Signature

Page.......

Date	Care Plan Ref. No.	Nursing Prescription	Signature

Figure 8.5: Examples of Headings for the Nursing Report

Page.......

Date	Nur./Orders Ref. No.	Observations/Report/Evaluation	Signature

Page.......

Date	Nur./Order Ref. No.	Nursing Report	Signature

to function effectively the pages will need holes on both sides if ring folders are used and completed assessment and nursing orders sheets placed in order towards the front of the file, while completed care plan and evaluation sheets are placed in order towards the back of the file.

This sounds complicated, but a brief experiment with some coloured sheets of paper headed with the different aspects of the documentation will clarify the scheme. What will emerge is the great difficulty of keeping the relevant entries about specific aspects of nursing adjacent to each other. To avoid a lot of repetitious writing it may be found helpful to plan into the documentation a page number and item number reference system.

The care plan will not use as many pages as the nursing orders and the nursing orders will not use as many pages as the report and evaluation record. This can lead to a muddle of pages in the folder and wasted time spent in hunting for the current entries.

Because the Nursing Report must contain a factual account of nursing done, both for current use and future reference, it is only by using a numbered reference system that a full account of nursing care given can be obtained for each care plan entry. The example of documentation in Appendix 4 shows how a number reference system can be planned into the documentation.

The main advantages of using a folder format for nursing documentation are that it has the potential to provide more space, it can be taken 'all of a piece' away from the storage point for recording or reference, it should be cheaper than cards and it is easier than cards to store with the patient's medical record on discharge.

A Card System for the Nursing Record

Most nurses are aware of what have come to be called Kardex® cards and holders. Several office suppliers now manufacture card holders and supply standard or specially printed cards for them.

It has been stated previously that success in implementing the Nursing Process depends, in part, on getting the documentaton right. Printed cards are more expensive than printed sheets of paper, so it is more important to get them right first time. This is because once the documentation has been accepted as the authorised record of nursing care given, mistakes in either the headings or the entries must not be blanked out with correcting fluid because of

Figure 8.6: An Extended Card for Documentation

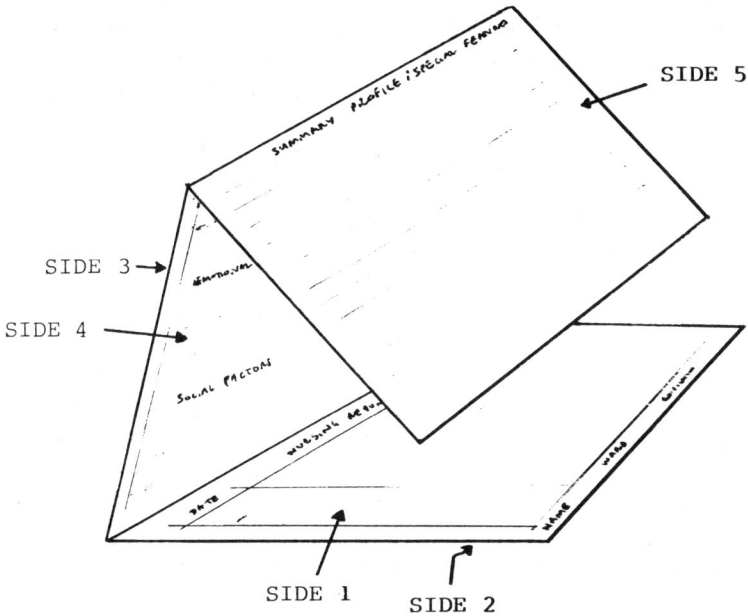

SIDE 5

SIDE 3

SIDE 4

SIDE 1 SIDE 2

legal implications.

In many hospitals the wards have been issued with 'Kardex' holders and cards for the traditional nursing reports and this makes it tempting to consider a card format for the Nursing Process record. Where the holders are for larger size cards it is well worth considering, but the smaller sizes do not provide enough space for adequate entries. Figure 8.6 illustrates the lay-out of a usefully extended Kardex-type card. Side 1 provides the first sheet of the 'report, observations and evaluation' and further cards or paper sheets can be inserted as the need arises. Side 2, which is the reverse side of Side 1, is not used. With Side 5 folded under, Side 3 provides the surface for the face sheet items. With Side 5 lifted, a long Side 4 is exposed for recording all the assessment information. The summary profile and any other information of importance is written on Side 5, which is visible when it is folded down and the card is open. Within the card holder, above the illustrated card there are slots for a further card which has to be used for the nursing care plan and nursing orders. These can be on either side of the card, but only one surface will be visible. When a folded card is used for a prolonged period it gets worn at the fold and can become detached, so it is necessary to write the patient's name and hospital number on the extension flap.

The choice of headings for the different parts of the card will depend on the same considerations as when deciding on the folder format sheets and readers are referred to Figures 8.1 to 8.5 above.

A card system has the advantage of being compact and transportable and easy to refer to. The disadvantages are that the space for entries is more limited, cards are more expensive than paper and when the number of cards increases with the patient's length of stay the slots of the holder tend to break. For additional cards, paper forms can be substituted, but although less expensive, they tend to fall out, and still cause the same problem of breaking the slots as numbers increase. Another disadvantage of a card system where the cards are kept in a special holder is that only one person can have access to the cards at a time, unless the cards are removed. One way round this problem is to punch holes in the cards and keep them in ring binders, but unless each patient's cards are in a separate binder this creates a problem of easily identifying a particular patient's nursing record. A further disadvantage is that, where special assessment, progress or observation charts are used as an adjunct to the nursing record, there is nowhere in the system to keep or store them.

When the documentation has been agreed and brought into use various other decisions have to be made. First there is the question of where to keep the nursing records. In some general hospitals, in order to serve the requirements of patient-centred care, the nursing record is kept by the patient's bed. In psychiatric hospitals the bed is certainly not the base for the majority of patients, so this is unlikely to be practicable, but records could be kept in a trolley in the day room if this was felt useful in deterring nurses from shutting themselves in the office while entering the records. Some district nurses leave their records in the patient's home and this could be a matter for debate among community psychiatric nurses.

The question of the accessibility of the nursing records leads on to the question of their confidentiality and this is more difficult to answer. If a patient has been able to contribute to the planning of his care and is consulted about the daily evaluations, there is perhaps no reason why any harm should be done if he reads his nursing record. It will challenge the nurse's accountability, but the greater difficulty arises from the possibility that if a patient has access to his own record, the chances are that other patients' records will be equally accessible. Nursing is a very public activity and in many wards the patients will know exactly how long a nurse spent talking to a particular patient, who is having modified insulin and who has been incontinent, etc. In some respects, knowing that care plans and reports may be read by the patients can improve the quality of care, so it is a question that bears consideration. If it is felt that it is an acceptable move to allow patients access to their nursing records then should patients raise confidential matters that they want kept secret, these can be referred to in a general way and the details kept with the medical notes.

Other questions that have to be answered about documentation concern the entries. Some discussion about who is to make the entries can be found in Chapter 7 on evaluation. This, and such matters as to whether night staff entries are in different coloured ink or particular safety aspects are underlined will have to be agreed policy.

There are coloured metal and plastic clips that can be slid on to the edge of cards or folders that, with agreed policy, can be used as markers to identify easily patients at special risk, or with particular needs or needing a specified nursing regime. As nurses implement the Nursing Process they meet various difficulties, but for those posed by documentation there are many manufacturers ready to explore these and suggest solutions.

This book started by saying that implementing the Nursing Process demanded change and one aspect of that change concerns evaluating and reviewing. If the philosophy of the Nursing Process itself is applied by nurses to their *implementation* of the Nursing Process, then they will be evaluating the effectiveness of the nursing and the documentation and hopefully answers to the questions posed will evolve with practice and experience.

9 GETTING STARTED

Getting started has to begin by being convinced. If, in reading this book, you have reached this point with some enthusiasm, then beginnings have to begin at the first stage, which is assessment. If you are working directly with patients choose someone you feel you do not know very well and while going about your work focus your attention on this person. If you have any spare minutes use him or her for interaction. After a few days start writing. First produce a general description of the patient and then jot down the facts you have noticed, concentrating on capabilities as well as disabilities. When you feel you really know this person and are not discovering anything new to record, try the checklist in Appendix 3 and see if you can give a factual appraisal for each item. If you find you are guessing for any item then explore further and check again. When you are satisfied, write out a tidy copy of your profile and assessment and try it out on your colleagues. Do they learn anything new about the patient? Are they left with any questions in their minds? Is your account factual or does it contain your value judgements?

If this has gone well, then proceed to the next patient, hopefully persuading some of your colleagues to try as well. Sometimes it is better for each nurse to take a different patient, but it can be more instructive for several nurses to assess one patient and compare notes. If it is done this way it must be remembered that this, as an exercise, is carried out over a period of time so that the patient chosen does not feel 'bombarded'.

While practising these assessment skills it is useful to identify whether any headings or questions on a list help in recording observations. It is from these experiments that useful contributions can be made when it comes to designing the documentation.

Once you feel confident at recording profiles and assessments and your colleagues are, hopefully, also practising and becoming skilled, then, in spare moments you can take one assessment and put into words the nursing that this patient needs. Again, this is better carried out with colleagues, but, if they are not willing, it is still useful to continue alone. You can make conscious the difficulties and your solutions so that you will be able to anticipate problems when the time does come to share your practised expertise with others.

It might happen that no one else does become interested but, by persevering to this stage, you will hopefully find that these conscious disciplines influence and enhance your own nursing practice, so the effort is not wasted. It also seems likely that, given time, orientation toward the Nursing Process will be required where you are working or you might move to another area where it is already accepted.

Continuing further without team support is very difficult, but experimenting with setting out Nursing Care plans and identifying what nursing is being carried out for the different patients can be useful. Although colleagues will be delivering much of the nursing care detailed in your plan, it is possible to identify something specific that you can carry out for one or several patients and then evaluate how effective it has been.

If you are a ward sister or charge nurse who wants to get started in a hospital that is not yet committed to the Nursing Process the initial stages have to be the same as for any individual nurse, but must involve all members of the nursing team. As each member becomes proficient at recording assessments and the team is able to agree on plans of care and has identified nursing activities and written some of them down as nursing actions, then it becomes important to discuss the format for documentation with nursing administrators and colleagues in other wards.

Nursing records are protected documents, which means they can be required for evidence in case of litigation or official enquiry. Because of this it is essential that there should be agreed policy and practice about the nursing records. For any team, this means that in the early stages of experimenting with the Nursing Process there will be a period while documents are being evolved where some of the writing will have to be duplicated for some and maybe all the patients. This is unfortunately inevitable until the Nursing Process documentation becomes the agreed legal record for the hospital or unit. It seems likely that, in the long term, this is preferable to the situation where untried documentation is 'imposed' before nursing teams are ready for it.

At any stage during the experimenting phase it is probably useful to plan a possible lay-out of headings, get some sheets duplicated and then try them out, making adjustments as necessary or convenient.

For nursing administrators, getting started means becoming convinced of the benefits of implementing the Nursing Process and then stimulating enthusiasm and encouraging nurses in their areas to get started as outlined above. It then means enabling interested nurses to meet with others in similar wards to share their successes and discuss their problems. It is important that nursing officers use their clinical expertise to monitor, guide, question and praise the efforts of the staff in their areas.

Eventually the documentation format will have to be agreed and sanctioned as the legal record. Participation in the various wards' experiments, discussion with colleagues and knowledge of the financial and storage implications should lead to satisfactory and useful documents. Where documents have already been designed and printed and their use imposed as hospital policy without adequate preparation, then nursing officers have the task of communicating an understanding of the philosophy of the Nursing Process. They will also need to provide an opportunity for their staff to assess and practise the skills required for the different stages of the Nursing Process and this is probably best done by setting up workshops. The number of workshops needed will vary, but old habits die hard and when new documentation is imposed without adequate tuition and help, the old ways are readily transferred and the new documents and the potential benefits of the Nursing Process by-passed. This can have the effect of the staff feeling they are being forced into a time-wasting exercise and therefore becoming increasingly resistant to change.

For nurse teachers, getting started means familiarising themselves with the philosophy of, and skills needed for, the Nursing Process. This should influence all their teaching, but particular help can be given to learners by setting the recording of patient profiles and assessments and the drawing up of nursing care plans as inter-block work. For theoretical teaching, getting started on the Nursing Process probably means being much more aware of what constitutes the activities of nursing and enabling learners to put into words what they actually do in the wards. The teacher can then help them identify to what extent those activities are likely to achieve stated objectives and then to encourage them to contribute possibly better, but realistic alternatives. For teaching in the clinical setting, getting started means generating and sustaining enthusiasm, taking an informed interest and supplying information and discussing problems raised with both learners and qualified staff. The nurse teacher may be invited to participate in care planning discussions and in such case should use directed questions to help the team work towards solutions, rather than offer advice.

If you are responsible for in-service training, getting started means identifying staff who show enthusiasm for, or interest in, the Nursing Process and organising workshops for them. Workshops, as well as providing information, must involve the participants in actually making assessments, drawing up care plans, detailing nursing activities and designing or familiarising themselves with documentation.

Study days which give only theoretical information and instruction appear to be less effective in imparting enthusiasm and encouraging nurses to get started. Indeed, they may be counter-productive in that participants are not required to check their level of skill and they can easily feel they are doing what is required already. Where this is the case, changes that are seen as unnecessary and time-consuming will be resisted.

For everyone, implementing the Nursing Process has to be a learned, internalised activity. No one can be directed 'to do it' without preparation and commitment. Once started it should carry its own momentum until, in the future, the Nursing Process will be so much part of nurse training and nursing that it will cease to need the designation and will become synonymous with nursing. When this happens nursing will have taken another step in its evolution.

POSTSCRIPT

Since most of this book was written, the Open University has published a learning package entitled 'A Systematic Approach to Nursing Care', which aims to provide nurses with a shared learning experience to enhance their understanding of the Nursing Process.

It has been written so that it can be applied to all fields of nursing. Most of the illustrative material relates to the general field but with a psychiatric nurse as facilitator the course can readily be related to the various spheres of psychiatric nursing. Readers of this book who have had their interest aroused but are left wishing to know more, are advised to contact their local School of Nursing Continuing Education Department, for further information about this Open University Course.

Further Reading

Altschul, A. T. 'Does good practice need good principles', *Nursing Times*, Vol. 80, No. 28 (1984), pp. 36—8, and No. 29, pp. 49—51
—— 'A systems approach to the Nursing Process'. *Journal of Advanced Nursing*, Vol. 3, No. 3 (1978), pp. 333—40
—— 'Use of the Nursing Process in psychiatric care'. *Nursing Times*, Vol. 73, No. 36 (1977), pp. 1412—3
Cormack, D. F. S. 'The Nursing Process: an application of the SOAPE model'. *Nursing Times*, Occasional Papers, Vol. 76, No. 9 (1980), pp. 37—40
Faulkner, A. 'Aye, there's the rub'. *Nursing Times*, Vol. 77, No. 8 (1981), pp. 332—6
Johnston, J. 'The Nursing Process and psychiatry'. *Nursing Mirror*, Vol. 158, No. 1 (1984), supplement
Jones, M. P. 'The Nursing Process in psychiatry'. *Nursing Times*, Vol. 76, No. 29 (1980), pp. 1273—5
Keane, P. 'The Nursing Process in a psychiatric context'. *Nursing Times*, Vol. 77, No. 28 (1981), pp. 1223—4
Stephenson, M. 'Problems remain'. *Nursing Mirror*, Vol. 158, No. 1 (1984), supplement
Stockwell, F. 'The Nursing Process in a psychiatric hospital'. *Nursing Times*, Vol. 78, No. 34 (1982), pp. 1441—2
Turner, J. 'It's not what you do . . .'. *Nursing Times*, Vol. 79, No. 4 (1983), p. 64.
Ward, M. 'The Nursing Process in psychiatry — the teacher's dilemma'. *Nursing Times*, Vol. 80, No. 25 (1984), pp. 46—8

APPENDIX 1: PHILOSOPHY, DEFINITION AND ACTIVITIES OF PSYCHIATRIC NURSING

A Philosophy of Psychiatric Nursing

Psychiatric nursing is an enabling and therapeutic process which recognises the uniqueness and worth of man who, when mentally ill, remains worthy of respect and entitled to dignity, and will have some or many aspects of behaviour capable of healthy functioning. It aims at bringing about by commitment, education and skilled intervention the realisation of the individual's optimum health and functioning, while affording comfort, support and protection where needed.

A Definition of Psychiatric Nursing

Psychiatric nursing is a complex, skilled, planned activity that aims, through teamwork and co-operation at: restoring the full healthy functioning of the mentally ill individual; minimising the affects of disabilities arising from illness or institutional care; protecting the individual from harm from within himself, from others or from the environment and ensuring maximum physical and psychological comfort.

A Summary of the Activities of Psychiatric Nursing

(1) Observation and recording observations.
(2) Ensuring that the physical needs for air, nutrition, hygiene and safety are met.
(3) Ensuring that the psychological needs for self-esteem, self-respect, individuality, contentment and spirituality are met.
(4) Providing opportunity for exercise and enhancement of all aspects of behaviour: physical, mental, emotional, social and spiritual.
(5) Limiting, preventing or compensating for disabilities and dysfunction.

(6) Carrying out prescribed treatments.
(7) Communicating in writing and verbally:
   Nurse ——— nurse
   Nurse ——— patient
   Nurse ——— medical staff
   Nurse ——— co-workers
   Nurse ——— relatives and friends of the patient
   Nurse ——— public at large

APPENDIX 2: AN ENHANCEMENT MODEL OF PSYCHIATRIC NURSING

This model sees the patient as a person with many innate and learned capacities who, through living, has grown, developed and acquired some or many skills and aptitudes, but who through suffering from mental illness becomes dependent in some degree on the help, support and care of others. It sees the nurse as a person who, primarily, identifies the strengths and capabilities of the patient, and devises strategies and opportunities to ensure these are exercised and enhanced. Secondarily but concurrently she uses her personal attributes and learned skills to ensure the patient's safety, and wellbeing, and to alleviate or minimise difficulties and disabilities, in accordance with medical philosophy and prescribed treatments.

The diagram in Figure 2.1 on p. 15 shows two individuals who meet on life's path in a nurse–patient relationship, each bringing to the encounter their unique personalities, their strengths and weaknesses and the totality of their experiences. The nurse and patient are given equal prominence to illustrate that in their common humanity neither is 'better' nor 'worse' than the other. The two meet as nurse and patient and through interaction get to know each other and build a bridge of trust between themselves. While this is happening they both contribute to the assessment and profile that will be recorded.

Throughout the subsequent nursing they both have to give and take from each other. Where the patient is very ill he will have to do more taking to begin with, but even so, if the nurse focuses on whatever strengths are there, this should have the effect of making him feel enhanced as a person.

The nurse will use her various skills to ensure that any prescribed treatment is carried out safely and with maximum benefit, and will utilise all the physical, social and recreational resources to enable the patient to participate and contribute safely and beneficially, whether at home or in a ward. Increasingly, as the patient becomes less dependent on the nurse, he should feel more a person and less a patient. This can be true even where illness is chronic or severe.

Both nurse and patient are living their lives during the period of the relationship, so, whatever happens between them becomes part of each one's life experience. Hopefully, there will be more positive factors than negative ones, and thus both participants will have good memories of a useful and happy encounter.

71

A relationship between a particular patient and a particular nurse does not occur in isolation, even in the community. The model takes account of the influence of other workers and other participants and indicates that they also contribute to all aspects of nursing while the individual nurse–patient relationship is ongoing.

APPENDIX 3: AN OUTLINE GUIDE FOR MAKING OBSERVATIONS OF PATIENTS

The following list provides a guide to the areas of an individual's behaviour which must be explored in order to evaluate his capabilities and difficulties so that the nurse can draw up a profile and assessment.

Do not use this uncritically as a checklist, but refer to it for reminders.

Capabilities		Associated Disabilities
Physical Capacities		*Incapacities*
Reflex	— Breathing	Lack of lung expansion
	Coughing	Effects of smoking
	Sneezing	
	Pulse	
	Blood pressure	
Swallowing	— Digestion	Over — or under — eating foraging
Elimination and	Excretion	Incontinence
Muscle activity	— Strength	Disease
	Co-ordination	Side effects of drugs
	Balance	Disuse atrophy and stiffness
	Gait	
	Joint mobility	

Activities of Daily Living	*Incapacities*
Hygiene	Lack of volition
Appetite	Lack of awareness
Exercise/Sleep	
Safety	
Warmth	
Toilet	

Sensory Capacities	*Incapacities*
Sight	All may be diminished or
Hearing	absent
Feeling	Illusions
Proprioception	Delusions
Balance	Hallucinations
Taste	
Smell	

73

Mental Capacities	*Incapacities*
Orientation	Preoccupation
Attention	May be unable to attend
Concentration	May be easily distracted
Verbal ability	Disorientation
Numerical ability	Failure to memorise
Reading	Limited recall: short-term
Writing	long-term
Memory: short-term	Neologisms
long-term	Thought block
Ideas — thinking	Apathetic — impulsive
Creativity	
Imagination	
Humour	
Volition/motivation	
Decision-making	
Insight	

Emotional Capacities	*Incapacities*
Capacity to experience emotions	Lack of affect
	Depression — elation
	Anxiety
Capacity to express emotions	Limited — excessive
	Inappropriate
Mental mechanisms	Attention seeking
	Paranoia
	Dissociation etc.

Social Capacities	*Social Incapacities*
Ability to initiate interaction — with whom? How often?	Abusive
Ability to be receptive to interaction — with whom? How often?	Aggressive
Awareness of social controls:	Ill-mannered
Manners	Inconsiderate
Conformity to norms, rules and routines	Isolated
Consideration	Depraved

Social Capacities — continued

Ability to communicate:
   Feelings
   Ideas
   Approval
Friendships

APPENDIX 4: A SUGGESTED ASSESSMENT NURSING CARE PLAN, NURSING ORDERS AND REPORT FOR THE EXAMPLE PATIENT IN CHAPTER 4

1. Assessment

DATE	ASSESSMENT PROFILE	SIGNATURE
11.2.80	June has taught English in a comprehensive school since qualifying seven years ago. She states she was well until her mother died ten months ago but with hindsight thinks she was ill before but was too busy to notice. Since then she had increasing pain, mostly in her back but sometimes 'inside', palpitations and weakness in her legs which prevents her working for or standing in class. She is convinced she is seriously ill because no one will tell her what is wrong and she sounds and looks apprehensive. She is articulate but mainly talks about herself. Her voice is flat and she expresses no emotion when talking about her mother. She looks after herself well, eating with encouragement and sleeping with prescribed hypnotics. She never relaxes into a chair and walks with a tense 'careful' gait. Full hip movement was observed as she got in and out of the bath. She is reluctant to participate or interact with other patients, usually sitting with an open book, yet very watchful and aware. She persistently engages nursing staff with questions or requests for Panadol for the aching pain. Physical observations: T. 36.6°C P. 92 R. 22 B/P 115/56 Weight 54.4 kg. Urine Sp.Gr. 1020 Acid N.A.D. Last period 24.1.80 (28 day cycle, sometimes irregular)	C. Clegg
13.2.80	A visiting friend said she was very active and sociable until her mother was ill and now she is like a different person.	C. Clegg

| NAME | HOSPITAL NO. | WARD | Page |

2. Nursing Care Plan

DATE	OBJECTIVES	NURSING PLAN	REVIEW DATE
10.2.80	1) To make her feel welcome	a) 'Time' from all nurses. b) Make her welcome in any ward activities she wishes to join in. c) Include in 'ward work' rota. Own choice of job to start with.	17.2.80
	2) To reduce anxiety level and physical symptoms	a) Identify episodes of increased anxiety and explore preceding stress factors b) Formal relaxation session daily. c) Teach about effects of tension on the body. d) Point out tension when observed and show how to 'let go'.	17.2.80
	3) To help her feel likeable	a) Identify nurse(s) who are most sympathetic and these to explore her strengths and abilities and organise activities where she can use them, individually or in a small group. b) See 1.a)	21.2.80
	4) To minimise complaints	a) Listen and explore sympathetically. b) Allow a rest on her bed for up to 1 hour. c) Discourage analgesics and hypnotics but refer to sister if insistent. d) Record sleeping pulse until thyroid function tests complete.	Daily

NAME	WARD	HOSPITAL NO.	Page

3. Nursing Orders

DATE	REF. NO. PAGE ITEM	NURSING ORDERS	RESPONSIBLE NURSE	SIGNA-TURE
11.2.80	1/1a	Chat interaction.	All staff	AS
	1/1 b & c 1/2 a–d 1/3 & 4	Encourage attendance at art workshop a.m. Relaxation after lunch. Key-worker role and observations.	St/N Platt	PP

NAME	WARD	HOSPITAL NO.	Page

4. Report

DATE	REF. NO. PAGE ITEM	OBSERVATIONS / REPORT / EVALUATION	SIGNATURE
11.2.80	1/1a	Uses nurse's attention to offload complaints. Refusing to talk to male staff.	⎫
	1/1b	Attended art unwillingly. Drew small flower slowly. Not helping in ward yet.	⎬ P. Platt
	1/2	Tense and restless all day, but no specific complaints.	⎭
	1/3 and 4	Relaxation had limited effect. P116 before and P108 after. Rapport very limited. More relaxed during art but resisted all other offers of occupation.	
11.2.80	1/4c	Offered Mogadon 5 mgs. Requested '2 tablets', which were given. Slept peacefully. Sleeping pulse at 3.15 a.m. 92/min. Drowsy this morning.	B. Briggs

NAME	WARD	HOSPITAL NO.	Page

INDEX